Beatrice Gehrmann
Wolf-Gerald Koch
Claus O. Tschirch
Helmut Brinkmann

Medicinal Herbs
A Compendium

Pre-publication
REVIEWS,
COMMENTARIES,
EVALUATIONS . . .

"**I**f you have ever been in a situation where you are drawing a blank on an herb's correct dose or a contraindication, you will now be able to find it in this book, which is designed as a quick fact-checker for the experienced herbal practitioner. You will probably end up having to buy more than one copy of this handy volume, because your friends and colleagues will walk off with yours."

David Edelberg, MD
Founder, American WholeHealth;
Author, *The Triple Whammy Cure*

"**M**edicinal Herbs: A Compendium is a one-of-a-kind synopsis of 200 commonly used medicinal herbs, which includes among other things, the common and Latin names of the herbs, a listing of the major uses of each herb, how to easily make preparations for use, plus contraindications and side effects. Most of the information is derived from books and reviews based primarily on the German experience, which is more extensive than from any other country. The book is simple, easy to use, and contains a wealth of information that should be beneficial to the consumer or others desiring a 'snapshot' of information on each herb. I highly recommend this very interesting compilation of herbal information."

Norman R. Farnsworth, PhD
Research Professor of Pharmacognosy and Distinguished University Professor, University of Illinois at Chicago, College of Pharmacy

The Haworth Herbal Press®
An Imprint of The Haworth Press, Inc.
New York • London • Oxford

Medicinal Herbs
A Compendium

THE HAWORTH HERBAL PRESS
Titles of Related Interest

Concise Handbook of Psychoactive Herbs: Medicinal Herbs for Treating Psychological and Neurological Problems by Marcello Spinella

Herbal Medicine: Chaos in the Marketplace by Rowena K. Richter

Botanical Medicines: The Desk Reference for Major Herbal Supplements, Second Edition by Dennis J. McKenna, Kenneth Jones, and Kerry Hughes

Typer's Tips: The Shopper's Guide for Herbal Remedies by George H. Constantine

Handbook of Psychotropic Herbs: A Scientific Analysis of Herbal Remedies for Psychiatric Conditions by Ethan B. Russo

Understanding Alternative Medicine: New Health Paths in America by Lawrence Tyler

Seasoning Savvy: How to Cook with Herbs, Spices, and Other Flavorings by Alice Arndt

Tyler's Honest Herbal: A Sensible Guide to the Use of Herbs and Related Remedies, Fourth Edition by Steven Foster and Varro E. Tyler

Tyler's Herbs of Choice: The Therapeutic Use of Phytomedicinals, Second Edition by James E. Robbers and Varro E. Tyler

Medicinal Herbs
A Compendium

Beatrice Gehrmann
Wolf-Gerald Koch
Claus O. Tschirch
Helmut Brinkmann

The Haworth Herbal Press®
An Imprint of The Haworth Press, Inc.
New York • London • Oxford

Published by

The Haworth Herbal Press, an imprint of The Haworth Press, Inc., 10 Alice Street, Binghamton, NY 13904-1580.

PUBLISHER'S NOTE
This book has been published solely for educational purposes and is not intended to substitute for the medical advice of a treating physician. Medicine is an ever-changing science. As new research and clinical experience broaden our knowledge, changes in treatment may be required. While many potential treatment options are made herein, some or all of the options may not be applicable to a particular individual. Therefore, the author, editor, and publisher do not accept responsibility in the event of negative consequences incurred as a result of the information presented in this book. We do not claim that this information is necessarily accurate by the rigid scientific and regulatory standards applied for medical treatment. **No warranty, expressed or implied, is furnished with respect to the material contained in this book. The reader is urged to consult with his/her personal physician with respect to the treatment of any medical condition.**

Revised and updated English edition of *Arzneidrogenprofile: Beratungsempfehlungen für die Pharmazeutische Praxis* © 2000 Deutscher Apotheker Verlag, Birkenwaldstrasse 44, 70191 Stuttgart, Germany.

Cover design by Marylouise E. Doyle.

Library of Congress Cataloging-in-Publication Data

Arzneidrogenprofile für die Kitteltasche. English.
 Medicinal herbs : a compendium / Beatrice Gehrmann . . . [et al.].
   p. ; cm.
 Includes bibliographical references.
 ISBN 0-7890-2530-2 (hard : alk. paper) — ISBN 0-7890-2531-0 (soft : alk. paper)
 1. Materia medica, Vegetable—Handbooks, manuals, etc. 2. Medicinal plants—Handbooks, manuals, etc. I. Gehrmann, Beatrice. II. Title.
 [DNLM: 1. Plants, Medicinal—Handbooks. 2. Phytotherapy—Handbooks. QV 735 A797m 2000a]
 RS164.A7913 2004
 615'.321—dc22
                                                                                    2004012972

CONTENTS

ABOUT THE AUTHORS

Beatrice Gehrmann is a pharmacist for Einhorn-Rats-Pharmacy in Husum, Germany. Dr. Gehrmann received her PhD in Pharmaceutical Biology/Pharmacognosy from Hamburg University. She is a member of the American Society of Pharmacognosy, the Society for Medicinal Plant Research, and Groupe Polyphénols. She is active in public pharmacy, research projects on medicinal plants at the Free University of Berlin, and has taught at different universities in Germany (Berlin, Leipzig, Hamburg). Dr. Gehrmann is the author of several scientific publications and compendia on medicinal herbs and pharmacognosy.

Wolf-Gerald Koch is a pharmacist at the Wartburg Pharmacy in Hamburg, Germany. Dr. Koch received his PhD in Pharmaceutical Biology/Pharmacognosy from Hamburg University. He is the head of a manufacturing and controlling group in the pharmaceutical industry. He is active in public pharmacy and the author of several scientific publications and compendia on medicinal herbs and pharmacognosy.

Claus O. Tschirch is a pharmacist at the "Gode Wind" Pharmacy in Hamburg, Germany. Dr. Tschirch received his PhD in Pharmaceutical Biology/Pharmacognosy from Hamburg University. He is a member of the German Pharmaceutical Society and the Society for Medicinal Plant Research. He is active in public pharmacy and the author of several scientific publications and compendia on medicinal herbs and pharmacognosy. Dr. Tschirch served in admission procedures in a hospital pharmacy.

Helmut Brinkmann, MD, DMD, is Head of the Department of Naturopathy and Head of the Department of Physical and Rehabilitative Medicine at Klinikum Nord (Ochsenzoll) in Hamburg, Germany. Dr. Brinkmann is a member of the Central Association of Physicians for Natural Treatment, the Society of Physicians for Therapeutic Fasting and Alimentation, and the Professional Association of Physicians for Physiotherapy and Physical Therapy. He is the author of several publications and is active in teaching.

Foreword

I am pleased to provide this brief foreword for *Medicinal Herbs: A Compendium*. Medicinal herbs have always played an important role in traditional medicine systems and are now playing increasingly important roles in Western medicine systems as well. This compedium, prepared in a concise and accurate manner, will be of great value for all English-speaking health professionals and consumers of herbal medicines. This book is timely and of special interest to both medical practitioners exercising phytotherapy and pharmacists. In much of the world, knowledge of and experience with medicinal herbs is superior to the current situation in the United States. Controversy abounds regarding efficacy, standardization, active ingredients, and potential toxicity or side effects. Clearly it will be many years before these issues are resolved, but the pharmacist remains well postioned to serve as a key expert in the area. Few have done more to promote a proper and accurate understanding of herbals than my predecessor, Dr. Varro (Tip) E. Tyler. The authors, in collaboration with Professor Tyler, and subsequently with his lovely wife, Ginny, have provided an important service in creating this compendium. I offer my hearty congratulations to them and best wishes to all who will benefit through its use.

John M. Pezzuto
Professor and Dean
Schools of Pharmacy, Nursing, and Health Sciences
Purdue University
West Lafayette, Indiana

Preface

In recent years, medicinal herbs and their preparation have been increasingly considered in the treatment of illness. The German compendium *Arzneidrogenprofile,* containing the profiles of about 200 commonly used medicinal herbs, was published in 2000. The aim of that compendium was to assist pharmacists by providing important information on medicinal herbs and their preparation in a succinct, easy-to-use form.

The choice of medicinal herbs to be profiled had to be subjective; the listed herbs were chosen after consideration of the data in the German Commission E monographs published in the *Bundesanzeiger,* the counterpart of the U.S. Federal Register, which have now been published in English translation by the American Botanical Council in Austin, Texas, as well as consideration of the data in the ESCOP (European Scientific Cooperation on Phytotherapy) monographs. Results of polls in Europe and North America regarding herbs and their uses and also the experiences of pharmacists were taken into consideration when choosing which medicinal herbs to profile.

The profiles of certain herbs important in European pharmacognosy but little known in North America were replaced by others that have importance for the North American medicinal herb market and according to the suggestions of Professor Varro E. Tyler.

The authors would like to point out that the profiles can provide only partial knowledge. Additional information should be taken from the bibliography at the end of the book.

Acknowledgments and Dedication

To our families, friends, colleagues, and former professors who are all in their very special ways interested in and encouraging our practical and theoretical work on medicinal herbs, phytomedicines, and phytotherapy: We are very grateful for their support and consistent help in so many ways.

We also wish to express special thanks to our German publishing house, the Deutscher Apotheker Verlag in Stuttgart, especially Sabine Körner, MA, and Eberhard Scholz, PhD.

Last but not least, we are deeply thankful to the late Professor Varro E. Tyler, PhD, ScD, who wholeheartedly supported the idea of translating and updating the German compendium *Arzneidrogen-profile* and offered to help edit it. Professor Tyler indeed was able, before his death in August 2001, to edit a large part of the compendium. For this reason, and because of his many years of experience and service in the field of European and American pharmacognosy, we sincerely wish to dedicate this compendium to his memory.

Profile Structure, Abbreviations, and Keys

HOW TO USE THE PROFILES

Medicinal Herb

Part used

Latin binomial AUTHOR

AA   **Area of Application**

The areas of application that are discussed are based on the reports of the German Commission E as published in the *Bundesanzeiger*. In addition, the following references were consulted and considered: R. Hänsel, K. Keller, H. Rimpler, and G. Schneider (Eds.), *Hagers Handbuch der Pharmazeutischen Praxis,* Fifth Edition (1992-1994); W. Blaschek, R. Hänsel, K. Keller, J. Reichling, H. Rimpler, and G. Schneider (Eds.), *Hagers Handbuch der Pharmazeutischen Praxis,* Fifth Edition, Supplements 2 and 3 (1998); N. G. Bisset and M. Wichtl, *Herbal Drugs and Phytopharmaceuticals* (2001); R. Braun (Ed.), *Standardzulassungen für Fertigarzneimittel* (2003) basic issue including fifteenth supplement; and various pharmacopeias including commentary in their current editions. Most of these herbs are named in the German Commission E monographs or in Chang et al. (1985, 1986), as well as in Tang and Eisenbrand (1992).

D   **Dosage**

For tea preparation, hot water is poured over the suggested quantity of medicinal herb and sieved after the proposed amount of time.

Example: 5 g/150 mL, 10-15 min, 1 cup 3 times/day

Divergence from this method of preparation, such as cold maceration, receives special consideration.

The necessary quantity of medicinal herbs is indicated in grams; in addition, the teaspoon dosage is mentioned, teaspoons having a capacity of about 4.0 to 4.5 mL of water. The amounts given were compared to the data cited by Wichtl (2002) and Braun (1997).

Preparations of herbs containing essential oils should always be covered during infusion, maceration, and so forth.

Due to possible microbial contamination, a cold maceration should be brought to a boil for a short time.

The dosage of other preparations is suggested if the use of herbal teas is not recommended.

For preparation of therapeutic baths, the amount of herb per 100 L water is reported. It is recommended to prepare the infusion using the whole herb amount and a smaller quantity of water in a separate container. After sieving, the infusion is poured into the bathtub, which can then be filled up with water of the desired temperature.

A   Application

Instructions for the duration of application and the necessity of consulting a medical practitioner are suggested.

C   Comments

This section provides information about the use of the herbs, their efficacy, and their safety, as well as particular risks. The traditional and/or folk medicinal use is mentioned in particular.

CI   Contraindications

Serious contraindications are listed in this section.

AE   Adverse Events

Important adverse events are listed and should be interpreted as follows:

Frequent:	> 10 percent
Occasional:	1-10 percent
Rare:	< 1 percent

Very rare: < 0.1 percent
Individual cases: without quantification

I   Interactions

Important and significant interactions are listed in this section.

The contents of the active principles of the medicinal herbs are not enumerated because such detailed information is beyond the scope of a compendium. More detailed data may be found in the works listed in the bibliography.

MEDICINAL HERB PROFILE KEY

Medicinal Herb

Part used

Latin binomial AUTHOR

AA   **Area of Application**

D   **Dosage**

A   **Application**

C   **Comments**

CI   **Contraindications**

AE   **Adverse Events**

I   **Interactions**

ABBREVIATIONS

approx.	approximately
CVI	chronic venous insufficiency
esp.	especially
g	gram
h	hour
L	liter
min	minute
mL	milliliter
NYHA	New York Heart Association
PMS	premenstrual syndrome
TCM	traditional Chinese medicine
V/V	volume/volume
WHO	World Health Organization
y	year
>	longer, greater than
<	shorter, less than
→	consequence
↑	increase, rise
↓	decrease

PICTOGRAMS KEY

 Tea or preparation to be taken with meals.
These instructions are not without exceptions, particularly for certain galenical preparations.

 Tea or preparation to be taken between meals.
These instructions are not without exceptions, particularly for certain galenical preparations.

 Tea or preparation to be taken 30-60 min before meals.
These instructions are not without exceptions, particularly for certain galenical preparations.

 Tea or preparation to be taken after meals.
These instructions are not without exceptions, particularly for certain galenical preparations.

 Dosage instructions and intervals must be strictly adhered to.

 Fluid intake must be sufficient.

Not to be used during pregnancy and nursing.

 Exposure to sunlight and UV radiation must be avoided.

 Drug has allergenic potential.

 Interaction between drug constituents and other drugs is possible.

 Efficacy has not been proven for the indications given here. Therapeutic use of the herb is not recommended because of the risks.

 Efficacy has not been proven for the claimed indications given here. Use of the herb is not associated with any known risks.

 Use only standardized extracts or commercial preparations.

PROFILES

Agrimony
Agrimoniae herba
Agrimonia eupatoria L.

AA: **Internal:** Mild, nonspecific, and acute diarrhea
Local: Inflammation of mouth, throat, and pharyngeal mucosa
External: Poultice for mild superficial skin inflammation

D: **Internal:** 1.5 g (1 teaspoon)/150 mL, 10-15 min, 1 cup 2-4 times/day
Local: Warm decoction used as gargle; for preparation, *see* INTERNAL
External: Poultice, freshly prepared, several times per day: 10 g/100 mL cold maceration, boil for a few minutes

A: For diarrhea > 2 days, with blood in stool or fever:
Please consult medical practitioner.

CI: Do not use for diarrhea in babies and infants.

AE: Unknown

I: Unknown

Angelica Root
Angelicae radix
Angelica archangelica L.

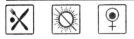

AA: Loss of appetite, feeling of fullness, flatulence, and minor gastrointestinal complaints

D: 2-4 g (1 teaspoon)/150 mL, 10 min, 1 cup 1-2 times/day before meals, daily dose 4.5 g
fluid extract (1:1): 1.5-3 g
tincture (1:5): 1.5 g
essential oil: 10-20 drops

A: Acute complaints > 1 week or recurring illness:
Please consult medical practitioner.

CI: Pregnancy; gastrointestinal ulcer

AE: Exposure to direct sunlight or intensive UV radiation may cause photosensitization; → skin inflammation possible

I: Unknown

Anise
Anisi fructus
Pimpinella anisum L.

AA: **Inhalation:** Bronchial congestion
      Internal: Bronchial congestion; dyspeptic complaints

D: **Inhalation:** 1.5 g (½ teaspoon), freshly crushed/150 mL, 10 min, 1 cup in the morning and/or in the evening
      Internal: 1.5 g freshly crushed/150 mL, 10 min, 1 cup in the morning and/or in the evening daily dose: 3 g; botanical products/preparations accordingly

A: Acute complaints > 1 week or recurring illness:
      Please consult medical practitioner.

C: Gustatory herbal drug; used as spice and in liqueur industries

CI: Pregnancy when eating fruits with very high amount of anethol; care for herbs with analytical certificate; allergy to anise, anethol

AE: Occasional allergic reactions affecting skin, airways, and gastrointestinal tract

I: Unknown

Arnica Flower/Leopard's Bane/Arnica Tincture
Arnicae flos, A. tinctura
Arnica montana L.

AA: Traumatic edema, hematoma, distortion, and contusion; rheumatic muscle and joint complaints; inflammation of mouth, throat, and pharyngeal mucosa, furunculosis; inflammation resulting from insect bite or sting, superficial vein inflammation

D: **External:** 3 g (4 teaspoons)/150 mL, 10-15 min
poultice: alcoholic tincture, 3-10 times diluted with water
mouthwash: alcoholic tincture, 10 times diluted with water

A: Acute complaints > 1 week or recurring illness:
Please consult medical practitioner.

C: Not for internal use due to risk of severe mucosal irritation (vomiting, diarrhea, mucosal bleeding) and myocardial paralysis as consequence of short-term stimulation of heart activity; cross-reacting allergy with other Asteraceae; frequent application may cause allergic contact dermatitis

CI: Allergy to arnica

AE: Long-term application and high concentration → edematous dermatosis, eczema; *see also* C

I: Unknown

Artichoke Leaf
Cynarae folium
Cynara scolymus L.

AA: Dyspeptic complaints, loss of appetite, lipid-lowering activity, hepatic stimulation

D: 2 g/150 mL, 5 min, 1 cup 3 times/day
daily dose: 6 g
single dose: dry extract, 500 mg

A: Acute complaints > 1 week or recurring illness:
Please consult medical practitioner.

C: Fresh leaves, freshly expressed plant sap/juice, and dry extract are used; for improving fat digestion; only commercial preparations containing standardized extracts are recommended.

CI: Do not use if obstructed biliary duct, gallstones exist;
→ risk of colic; avoid if known allergy to artichoke and other Asteraceae/members of daisy family

AE: Skin contact causes moderate sensitization;
allergic reactions possible, especially in those processing the plant professionally ("on-the-job" contact)

I: Unknown

Ashwagandha

Withaniae somniferae radix
Withania somnifera DUNAL

AA: Ayurvedic medicine: tonic; adaptogenic activity

A: Acute complaints > 1 week or recurring illness:
Please consult medical practitioner.

C: Efficacy not proven; cannot be considered a useful adaptogen/tonic

CI: Unknown

AE: Unknown

I: Unknown

Astragalus
Astragali radix
Astragalus membranaceus (FISCH.) BGE.
var. *mongolicus* (BGE.) HSIAO

⊙

AA: Immunostimulating. Used in Chinese medicine as a tonic; further: edema, renal inflammations, diabetes mellitus, viral hepatitis

A: Acute complaints > 1 week or recurring illness:
Please consult medical practitioner.

C: Variety of indications and therapeutic effects; efficacy not yet proven

CI: Unknown

AE: Unknown

I: Unknown

Avocado Oil
Avocado oleum
Persea americana MILL.

AA: Ingredient in so-called natural cosmetics for skin care; moisturizes and smooths dry and scaly skin

C: Do not mix different batches of oils.

CI: Known allergy to preparations containing avocado oil

AE: Unknown

I: Unknown

Balm Leaf/Lemon Balm/Melissa
Melissae folium
Melissa officinalis L.

AA: Initial nervous insomnia, improving sleep, functional gastro-intestinal complaints; also applied in pediatrics

D: 1.5-4.5 g (3-7 teaspoons)/150 mL, 10-15 min, 1 cup several times/day

A: Acute complaints > 1 week or recurring illness: Please consult medical practitioner.

C: Combinations with other sedative and/or carminative effective herbal drugs may be useful.

CI: Unknown

AE: Unknown

I: Unknown

Barbados or Curaçao Aloe
Aloe barbadensis
Aloe barbadensis MILL.

Cape Aloe
Aloe capensis
Aloe ferox MILL.

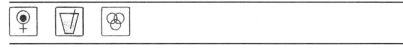

AA: Constipation

D: Single dose: 50 mg pulverized aloe in the evening;
daily dose: 50-200 mg pulverized aloe, equivalent to 20-30 mg hydroxyanthraquinone derivatives. The individual correct dosage is the lowest that is necessary to obtain a smooth stool.

A: Duration of application: short-term therapy (maximum 1-2 weeks).
Please consult medical practitioner.

C: Long-term application may cause intensification of digestive disorder. Nutrition may be enriched by vegetable fibers; ensure sufficient fluid intake and body movement.

CI: Intestinal blockage; acute inflammatory intestinal illness (Crohn's disease, ulcerative colitis, appendicitis); abdominal pain of unknown cause; children < 12 y; pregnancy and lactation

AE: Individual cases of gastrointestinal cramping; frequent and long-term application or overdosage may lead to loss of electrolytes (potassium), albuminuria, hematuria

I: Deprivation of potassium → cardioactive glycosides ↑, influences the effect of antiarrhythmics

Bearberry Leaf
Uvae-ursi folium
Arctostaphylos uva-ursi (L.) SPRENGEL

AA: Inflammation of urinary tract and catarrh of bladder and renal pelvis

D: Single dose: 3 g (1-2 teaspoons)/150 mL, equivalent to 100-210 mg hydroquinone derivatives, boil for 15 min; cold maceration 6-12 h, 1 cup 3-4 times/day,
daily dose: 10-12 g, equivalent to 400-800 mg hydroquinone derivatives;
fluid extract: 2 g; dry extract: 0.4 g

A: Preparations and botanical products containing arbutin not > 1 week and maximum 5 times/year

C: Disinfectant effect of hydroquinone, released in urinary tract at pH > 7 → urine at pH > 7 (e.g., take with sodium bicarbonate)

CI: Pregnancy, lactation, children < 12 y

AE: Persons with sensitive stomach and children: nausea and vomiting possible

I: Substances that acidify urine → antibacterial effect ↓

Bilberry/Blueberry

Myrtilli fructus
Vaccinium myrtillus L.

AA: **Internal:** Nonspecific acute diarrhea, especially in mild cases of enteritis in infants
Local: Mild inflammation of mouth, throat, and pharyngeal mucosa

D: **Internal:** 10 g (2 teaspoons) crushed herbs/150 mL, 10 min, cold maceration 2h, 1 cup several times/day
Local: 10 percent infusion

A: For diarrhea lasting > 3-4 days:
Please consult medical practitioner.

C: Fresh bilberries are mildly laxative when consumed in excess.

CI: Unknown

AE: Unknown

I: Unknown

Bilberry Leaf/Blueberry Leaf
Myrtilli folium
Vaccinium myrtillus L.

AA: Astringent and antidiarrheal; enhancement of metabolism; complaints of gastrointestinal tract, kidney, derivative urinary tract; antidiabetic; antirheumatic

C: Efficacy not proved; therapeutic use not justified
Risks: high dosage and long-term application may cause chronic intoxication.
(animal experiments showed cachexia, anemia, and jaundice)

Birch Leaf
Betulae folium
Betula pubescens EHRH., *B. pendula* ROTH.

☒	▽

AA: Cleansing/irrigation therapy with bacterial and inflammatory illness of derivative/efferent urinary tract, specifically renal calculus and gravel; supportive therapy for rheumatic conditions

D: 2-3 g (2-3 teaspoons)/150 mL, 15 min,
1 cup 3-4 times/day freshly prepared between meals

A: Acute complaints > 1 week or recurring illness:
Please consult medical practitioner.

C: Ensure sufficient fluid intake, minimum 2 L/day

CI: Not useful for dehydration or edema due to reduced heart and renal activity

AE: Unknown

I: Unknown

Bitter Orange Peel
Aurantii pericarpium
Citrus aurantium L. ssp. *aurantium*

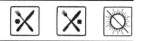

AA: Loss of appetite, digestive disorders,
feeling of fullness, bloating, and flatulence

D: 2 g (½ teaspoon)/150 mL, 10-15 min,
1 cup 2-3 times/day,
appetite enhancer → before meals,
digestive disorders → after meals

A: Acute complaints > 1 week or recurring illness:
Please consult medical practitioner.

C: Gustatory herb; component of gingerbread, vin brulé (mulled
wine) spice

CI: Unknown

AE: Photosensitization possible, particularly for persons with fair
skin

I: Unknown

Black Cohosh
Cimicifugae rhizoma
Cimicifuga racemosa (L.) NUTT.

AA: Menopausal complaints, neurovegetative PMS and dysmenorrhea

D: Single dose: 1 g, 5-10 min,
1 cup 3 times/day,
daily dose: extract (ethanol/water 40-60 percent [V/V], isopropanol/water 60 percent [V/V]), 10 mg equivalent to at least 40 mg herbal drug

A: Acute complaints > 1 week or recurring illness:
Please consult medical practitioner.

C: Herbal teas unusual, occasionally part of "women's teas"; commercial preparations containing standardized extracts are recommended.

CI: Pregnancy, lactation; patients being treated for hormone-dependent (estrogenic) tumors should avoid the herb.

AE: Occasional indigestion

I: Unknown

Black Knotweed/Hogweed
Polygoni avicularis herba
Polygonum aviculare L.

AA: **Internal:** Catarrh of respiratory tract
Local: Inflammation of mouth, throat, and pharyngeal mucosa

D: **Internal:** 1.5 g (1 teaspoon)/150 mL,
cold maceration, heat to boiling point, 5-10 min,
1 cup 3-5 times/daily,
daily dose: 4-6 g
Local: Gargle and cleansing; for dosage *see* INTERNAL

A: Acute complaints > 1 week or recurring illness:
Please consult medical practitioner.

CI: Unknown

AE: Unknown

I: Unknown

Black/European Elder Flower
Sambuci flos
Sambucus nigra L.

AA: Catarrh of respiratory tract, dry cough; treatment of febrile common cold as diaphoretic

D: 3-4 g (2-3 teaspoons)/150 mL, 5-10 min,
1-2 cups, several times/day, as hot as possible, especially during second half of day,
daily dose: 10-15 g

A: Acute complaints > 1 week or recurring illness:
Please consult medical practitioner.

CI: Unknown

AE: Unknown

I: Unknown

Blackberry Leaf
Rubi fruticosi folium
Rubus fruticosus L.

☒

AA: **Internal:** Mild, nonspecific, and acute diarrhea
Local: Mild inflammation of mouth, throat, and pharyngeal mucosa

D: **Internal:** 1.5 g (1-2 teaspoons)/150 mL, 10-15 min,
1 cup 2-3 times/day between meals,
daily dose: 2-5 g
Local: Gargle and cleansing; for dosage *see* INTERNAL

A: For diarrhea > 3-4 days:
Please consult medical practitioner.

CI: Unknown

AE: Unknown

I: Unknown

Blackthorn Flower

Pruni spinosae flos
Prunus spinosa L.

AA: Common cold, respiratory tract complaints; to support treatment for renal and bladder complaints/disturbances, prophylaxis and treatment of gastric spasms, flatulence, intestinal complaints, gastric weakness/sensitive stomach

D: 1-2 g (1 teaspoon)/150 mL, 5-10 min,
1 cup 1-2 times/day, or 2 cups in the evening

A: Acute complaints > 1 week or recurring illness:
Please consult medical practitioner.

C: Efficacy not proven;
no risks,
safe when consumed as a beverage and used as indicated

CI: Unknown

AE: Unknown

I: Unknown

Blackthorn Fruit
Pruni spinosae fructus
Prunus spinosa L.

AA: Inflammation of mouth, throat, and pharyngeal mucosa; localized gargling treatment

D: Gargle and cleansing:
2 g (1 teaspoon)/150 mL, 10-15 min,
gargle, cleanse 2 times/day,
daily dose: 2-4 g

A: Acute complaints > 1 week or recurring illness:
Please consult medical practitioner.

CI: Unknown

AE: Unknown

I: Unknown

Blessed Thistle/Holy Thistle
Cnici benedicti herba
Cnicus benedictus L.

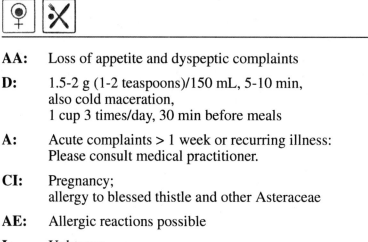

AA: Loss of appetite and dyspeptic complaints

D: 1.5-2 g (1-2 teaspoons)/150 mL, 5-10 min,
            also cold maceration,
            1 cup 3 times/day, 30 min before meals

A: Acute complaints > 1 week or recurring illness:
            Please consult medical practitioner.

CI: Pregnancy;
            allergy to blessed thistle and other Asteraceae

AE: Allergic reactions possible

I: Unknown

Blond Psyllium Husk/Seed/
Indian Plantago Husk/Seed/
Ispaghula Husk/Seed
Plantaginis ovatae testa/semen
Plantago ovata FORSK.

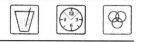

AA: Habitual constipation; illnesses which require facilitated bowel movement with smooth stool, e.g., anal fissures, hemorrhoids, after rectal-anal operations, pregnancy; supportive therapy for diarrhea and irritable bowel

D: 5-10 g dry seed (1-2 teaspoons)/150 mL, allow to soak,
200 mL fluid intake afterward,
daily intake: 4-20 g

A: For diarrhea > 3-4 days:
Please consult medical practitioner.

C: 30-60 min interval from intake of meals and other medication; ensure sufficient fluid intake, minimum 2 L/day

CI: Pathological narrowing of gastrointestinal tract,
inflammatory illness of gastrointestinal tract
→ risk of irritation and spasms; risk of intestinal blockage; diabetes mellitus difficult to regulate

AE: Rare hypersensitivity reactions

I: Simultaneous medication → absorption ↓;
insulin-dependent diabetes → dose of insulin ↓

Boldo Leaf
Boldo folium
Peumus boldus MOL.

AA: Mild cramping and gastrointestinal disturbances, dyspeptic complaints

D: 1-2 g (1-2 teaspoons)/150 mL, 10-15 min,
1 cup 2-3 times/day,
daily intake: 3-4.5 g

A: Acute complaints > 1 week or recurring illness:
Please consult medical practitioner.

C: Gallstones: only with medical advice
The essential oil and leaf distillates should not be used due to the high concentration of ascaridol.

CI: Biliary duct closure; severe hepatic disease

AE: Unknown

I: Unknown

Buckbean/Bogbean
Menyanthes folium, Trifolii fibrini folium
Menyanthes trifoliata L.

AA: Loss of appetite, dyspeptic complaints; bitter → gastric juice secretion ↑

D: 0.5-1 g fine cut (1 scant teaspoon)/150 mL, 5-10 min, also cold maceration, ½ cup before meals, unsweetened, 3 times/day, daily intake: 1.5-3 g

A: Acute complaints > 1 week or recurring illness: Please consult medical practitioner.

CI: Diarrhea, dysentery, colitis

AE: Overdose may cause stomach irritation, vomiting, diarrhea

I: Unknown

Buckthorn

Rhamni cathartici fructus
Rhamnus cathartica L.

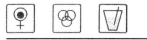

AA: Constipation

D: 2-5 g (1 teaspoon)/150 mL, 10-15 min,
1 cup in the morning and/or in the evening,
daily dose: maximum 5 g.
The individual correct dosage is the lowest that is necessary
to obtain smooth stool.

A: Duration of application: short-term therapy (maximum 1-2
weeks).
Please consult medical practitioner.

C: Long-term application may cause intensification of digestive
disorder. Nutrition may be enriched by vegetable fibers;
ensure sufficient fluid intake and body movement.
Use during pregnancy and lactation only with medical advice.

CI: Twisting of the intestines; acute inflammatory intestinal
illness (Crohn's disease, ulcerative colitis, appendicitis); abdominal pains of unknown origin;
children < 12 y; pregnancy and lactation

AE: Individual cases of gastrointestinal complaints with cramps;
frequent and long-term application or overdose may lead to
loss of electrolytes (potassium), albuminuria, hematuria

I: Deprivation of potassium → effect of cardioactive glycosides
↑, influences the effect of antiarrhythmics

Buckwheat Herb
Fagopyri herba
Fagopyrum esculentum MOENCH

AA: Chronic venous insufficiency (CVI); venous congestion, varicose vein formation

D: Approx. 2 g (2 teaspoons)/150 mL, 10-15 min,
1 cup 2-3 times/day for 4-8 weeks

A: Acute complaints > 1 week or recurring illness:
Please consult medical practitioner.

C: Efficacy with CVI proved by double-blind study; efficacy with venous congestion, varicose vein formation not proven

CI: Unknown

AE: In animals large amounts of fresh buckwheat herb may evoke phototoxicosis because of photosensitization by naphthodianthrone

I: Unknown

Bugleweed/Gypsywort
Lycopi herba
Lycopus europaeus L., *L. virginicus* L.

$\boxed{\circledgg}$

AA: Mild thyroid hyperfunction with disturbances of the vegetative nervous system; tension and pain in the breast (mastodynia)

D: 0.5-1 g (1 teaspoon)/150 mL, 10 min,
1 cup 2 times/day,
daily dose: 1-2 g

A: Acute complaints > 1 week or recurring illness:
Please consult medical practitioner.

C: Dosage is individual and varies depending on the symptom complex, age, and body weight.

CI: Thyroid gland hypofunction, euthyroid struma

AE: Long-term application and/or higher doses
→ enlargement of the thyroid; after terminating treatment →
rebound phenomenon may occur with increased TSH secretion and prolactin secretion as well as an increase of the hyperthyroid symptom complex and mastodynia

I: No simultaneous administration of thyroid hormones to depress the goitrogenic effect;
administration of *Lycopus* preparations disturbs the administration of diagnostic procedures with radioactive isotopes.

Burdock/Great Burdock
Bardanae radix
Arctium lappa L.

AA: **Internal:** Complaints of gastrointestinal tract
         External: Scaly skin, psoriasis, and seborrhea of scalp;
         eczema and to promote wound healing

D: **Internal:** 2.5 g (1 teaspoon)/150 mL, cold maceration,
         if necessary store for several hours, boil up to 1 h,
         1 cup 1-2 times/day
         External: Burdock fatty oil, hair oil as ointment,
         diluted with peanut oil 1:10

A: Acute complaints > 1 week or recurring illness:
         Please consult medical practitioner.

C: Efficacy not proven; no risks

CI: Hypersensitivity to Asteraceae

AE: Unknown

I: Unknown

Butcher's-Broom/Box Holly
Rusci aculeati rhizoma
Ruscus aculeatus L.

AA: Supportive therapy for CVI complaints such as heavy and painful legs, nocturnal calf pain, pruritus, and swelling; also supportive therapy for hemorrhoidal complaints such as pruritus and burning

D: Daily dose: 7-11 mg total ruscogenin

A: Acute complaints > 1 week or recurring illness:
Please consult medical practitioner.

C: Herbal teas unusual, commercial preparations containing standardized extracts are recommended.

CI: Unknown

AE: Very rarely, stomach complaints and nausea

I: Unknown

Calamus/Sweet Flag
Calami rhizoma
Acorus calamus L.

AA: **Internal:** Stomachic and carminative with digestive disorders, gastritis, and against ulcers
Local: Inflammation of mouth, throat, and pharynx

D: **Internal:** 1-1.5 g (½ teaspoon)/150 mL, 3-5 min,
also cold maceration, 30 min,
heat to boiling point before drinking,
1 cup with meals 3 times/day
Local: Gargle and cleansing; for preparation *see* INTERNAL

A: Acute complaints > 1 week or recurring illness:
Please consult medical practitioner.

C: No long-term use because of potential carcinogenocity due to
ß-asarone;
use diploid *Acorus calamus* race (ß-asarone free); analytical
certificate of herbal drug

CI: Pregnancy

AE: *See* C, carcinogenocity not clarified

I: Unknown

Calendula/Marigold Flower
Calendulae flos
Calendula officinalis L.

AA: **Internal:** Stomach complaints, gastrointestinal ulcers, gastritis and spasms of the gastrointestinal tract
Local: Inflammation of mouth, throat, and pharyngeal mucosa
External: Skin inflammations, wounds, to promote wound healing, ulcus cruris (ulceration on the lower leg)

D: **Internal:** 1-4 g (3-12 teaspoons)/150 mL, 10 min,
1 cup up to 3 times/day
Local: 2 g (6 teaspoons)/150 mL, 10 min,
gargle and cleanse several times/day
External: Poultice, dosage *see* LOCAL;
in ointments: 2-5 g/100 g ointment

A: Acute complaints > 1 week or recurring illness:
Please consult medical practitioner.

C: Used as ornamental herb;
warning: homemade ointments, using grease (lard) and tallow as a base → storage life ↓

CI: Known hypersensitivity to Asteraceae

AE: Sensitization possible (Asteraceae)

I: Unknown

Caraway
Carvi fructus
Carum carvi L.

AA: Dyspeptic conditions such as mild complaints of gastrointestinal tract, flatulence, and feeling of fullness as well as nervous heart-stomach troubles

D: 1-5 g (1 teaspoon) freshly crushed/150 mL,
10-15 min covered;
adults: 1 cup 1-3 times/day, daily dose: 1.5-6 g;
babies: adult dose, diluted 1:1 with freshly boiled water

A: Acute complaints > 1 week or recurring illness:
Please consult medical practitioner.

C: Aromatic and flavor-enhancing herb;
used as spice and in liqueur industries

CI: Unknown

AE: Unknown

I: Unknown

Cardamom

Cardamomi fructus
Elettaria cardamomum (L.) MATON

AA: Loss of appetite, dyspeptic complaints

D: 0.5-1 g (1/3 teaspoon)/150 mL, 10 min,
1 cup when required,
daily dose: 1-2 g

A: Acute complaints > 1 week or recurring illness:
Please consult medical practitioner.

C: Aromatic and flavor-enhancing herb;
ingredient in gingerbread

CI: Gallstones: use only with medical advice

AE: Unknown

I: Unknown

Carline Thistle
Carlinae radix
Carlina acaulis L.

AA: **Internal:** Atonic gastritis, inflammation of bilary ducts, dyspeptic complaints; febrile common cold
External: Dermatosis, wounds, ulcer

D: **Internal:** 1-3 g (1 teaspoon)/150 mL, boil for 10 min, steep for 30 min,
1 cup, 3 times/day between meals
External: 30 g (10 teaspoons)/1 L, boil for 10 min, infuse for 30 min, for pain relief and cleansing

A: Acute complaints > 1 week or recurring illness:
Please consult medical practitioner.

C: Efficacy not proven; component of Swedish bitters

CI: Unknown

AE: Unknown; higher doses → vomiting, diarrhea

I: Unknown

Cascara Sagrada/Sacred Bark/Chittem Bark
Rhamni purshiani cortex
Frangula purshiana (DC.) COOP.

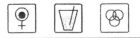

AA: Constipation

D: Up to 2 g (1 teaspoon)/150 mL, 10-15 min,
1 cup (freshly brewed) in the morning and/or in the evening,
daily dose: 20-30 mg hydroxyanthraquinone derivatives.
The individual correct dosage is the lowest that is necessary
to obtain a smooth stool.

A: Duration of application: short-term therapy (maximum 1-2
weeks).
Please consult medical practitioner.

C: Long-term application may cause intensification of digestive
disorder. Nutrition may be enriched by vegetable fibers;
ensure sufficient fluid intake and body movement.

CI: Intestinal blockage; acute inflammatory intestinal illness
(Crohn's disease, ulcerative colitis, appendicitis); abdominal
pains of unknown cause;
children < 12 y; pregnancy and lactation

AE: Individual cases of gastrointestinal cramping; frequent and
long-term application or overdose may lead to loss of electrolytes (potassium), albuminuria, hematuria

I: Deprivation of potassium → effect of cardioactive glycosides
↑, influences the effect of antiarrhythmics

Cat's Claw/Uña de Gato
Uncaria tomentosa radix
Uncaria tomentosa (WILLD.) DC.

AA: Immunostimulating; in Peruvian traditional medicine: as an anti-inflammatory, contraceptive, and cytostatic remedy

D: 3g (2 teaspoons)/150mL, 10 min, up to 1L/day

A: Acute complaints > 1 week or recurring illness:
Please consult medical practitioner.

C: Efficacy not yet proven.
Note: mixtures of specific chemotypes unsuitable for immunomodulating therapy

CI: Unknown

AE: Unknown

I: Unknown

Cayenne Pepper/Chilies/
Tabasco Pepper
Capsici fructus acer
Capsicum frutescens L.

AA:　**External:** painful muscular tension in the cervicobrachial range as well as in vertebral column; in folk medicine, internally for gastrointestinal disorders and seasickness

D:　Ointment: 0.02-0.05 percent capsaicinoides
Liniment: 0.005-0.01 percent capsaicinoides
Plaster: 10-40 µg/cm^2 capsaicinoides

A:　**External:** effective only after repeated application;
4-5 times/day for several weeks.
Internal application should be limited to 2 days; should only be used again after 2 weeks.

C:　No additional heat treatment
Capsicum preparations have strong mucosal irritation potential → Keep away from eyes

CI:　Previously damaged skin; hypersensitivity to capsicum preparations

AE:　Rare cases of hypersensitivity reactions

I:　Unknown

Chamomile/German Chamomile Flower
Matricariae flos
Matricaria recutita L.

AA: **Inhaled:** Inflammation and irritation of respiratory tract
Internal: Inflammation and irrigation of gastrointestinal tract
External: Inflammation of skin and mucosa, anal and genital inflammation
Local: Inflammation of skin and mucosa, of oral/mouth cavity and gingiva

D: **Inhaled:** Steam bath: Approx. 6 g (6 teaspoons)
Internal: 3 g (3 teaspoons)/150 mL, 5-10 min,
1 cup 3-4 times/day
External: Ointment (3-10 percent),
therapeutic bath: 50 g/10 L
Local: Gargle and cleansing (infusion 3-10 percent)
several times/day

A: Acute complaints > 1 week or recurring illness:
Please consult medical practitioner.

C: Do not use infusion ophthalmologically.

CI: Hypersensitivity to Asteraceae;
no local application with extensive skin lesions;
therapeutic full baths with fevers and infectious diseases, cardiac insufficiency Stage III-IV (NYHA), hypertonia Stage IV (WHO): only after consulting medical practitioner

AE: Unknown

I: Unknown

Chaste Tree
Agni casti fructus
Vitex agnus-castus L.

AA: Menstrual irregularities, menstrual disorder due to corpus luteum insufficiency, PMS, mastodynia

D: Commercial preparations according to package insert, daily dose: 30-40 mg herbal extract (water/ethanol); amenorrhea, oligomenorrhea:
40-45 drops once/day for 6 weeks;
fertility disturbance, PMS:
40 drops once/day for 3 cycles;
fluid extract: 1-2 g daily

A: Swollen breasts, menstrual cycle disturbances:
please consult medical practitioner for diagnosis.

C: Herbal teas unusual; commercial preparations containing standardized extracts are recommended.

CI: Pregnancy, lactation

AE: Itching, urticarious exanthem possible

I: Unknown

Chicory/Succory
Cichoriae herba et radix
Cichorium intybus L.

AA: Lack of appetite, dyspeptic complaints

D: Up to 2 g (1 teaspoon)/150 mL, 10 min,
1 cup 2 times/day,
daily dose: 3 g

A: Acute complaints > 1 week or recurring illness:
Please consult medical practitioner.

C: Also used as coffee substitute

CI: Allergy to Asteraceae; for gallstones: use only with medical
advice.

AE: Very rare cases of allergic skin irritation

I: Unknown

Chinese/Korean Ginseng Root
Ginseng radix
Panax ginseng C. A. MEY.

AA: Tonic for weariness, fatigue, weakness, reduced efficiency, and ability to concentrate as well as during convalescence

D: Tea: 3 g (1 teaspoon)/150 mL, 5-10 min, covered,
1 cup 1-3 times/day,
daily dose in preparations: 1-2 g
(minimum 10 mg ginsenosides)

A: Usually up to 3 months,
repeated application possible;
for persistent complaints,
Please consult medical practitioner.

C: Also commercial preparations containing standardized extracts

CI: Unknown

AE: Unknown

I: Unknown

Cinnamon Bark/Ceylon Cinnamon
Cinnamomi ceylanici cortex
Cinnamomum ceylanicum BLUME, *C. verum* J. S. PRESL.

Chinese Cassia/Cassia
Cinnamomi cassiae cortex
Cinnamomum aromaticum NEES.

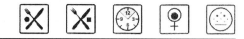

AA: Lack of appetite, dyspeptic complaints

D: 0.5-1 g (1/3 teaspoon)/150 mL, 10 min,
1 cup 2-4 times/day with meals
appetizer: 30 min before meal
gastrointestinal complaints: after meals,
daily dose 2-4 g
or 0.05-0.2 g essential oil,
equivalent to 2 drops 3 times/day

A: Acute complaints > 1 week or recurring illness:
Please consult medical practitioner.

C: Aromatic and flavor-enhancing herb;
ingredient in gingerbread

CI: Pregnancy; hypersensitivity to cinnamon and Balm of Peru

AE: Frequent allergic skin and mucosa irritations

I: Unknown

Cloves/Clove Oil

Caryophylli flos, C. aetheroleum
Syzygium aromaticum (L.) MERR. et L. M. PERRY

AA: **Local:** Essential oil: Inflammatory variations of mouth, throat, and pharyngeal mucosa; in dentistry as local analgesic and antiseptic
Internal: In combination with other herbs as stomachic and carminative

D: **Local:** Dentistry: essential oil, undiluted, mouthwash: 1-5 percent essential oil

A: Acute complaints > 1 week or recurring illness:
Please consult medical practitioner.

C: Aromatic and flavor-enhancing herb; ingredient of ginger-bread, vin brulé (mulled wine) spice

CI: Unknown

AE: Essential oil, undiluted, may cause tissue irritation; allergic skin and mucosa reactions possible

I: Unknown

Coltsfoot Leaf/Tussilago Leaf
Farfarae folium
Tussilago farfara L.

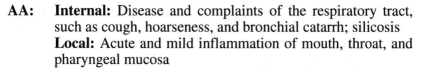

AA: **Internal:** Disease and complaints of the respiratory tract, such as cough, hoarseness, and bronchial catarrh; silicosis
Local: Acute and mild inflammation of mouth, throat, and pharyngeal mucosa

D: **Internal:** 1.5 g (1 teaspoon)/150 mL, 10-15 min,
1 cup 3-4 times/day,
daily dose: 4.5-6 g
Local: Gargle; for preparation *see* INTERNAL

A: Do not use > 4-6 weeks/year

C: Avoid long-term application: pyrrolizidine alkaloids are carcinogenic. Even traces (10 μg/day internally) may be harmful, only use certified herbs
Avoid herbs collected in the wild

CI: Pregnancy, lactation; hypersensitivity to Asteraceae

AE: Unknown

I: Unknown

Comfrey Leaf/Comfrey Herb
Symphyti folium, S. herba
Symphytum officinale L.

AA: Contusions, muscle strains, bruises, and sprains; stimulation of bone healing

D: Preparations for external use 5-20 percent,
         see also COMFREY ROOT

A: Duration of application: maximum 4 weeks/year

C: Only externally on intact skin; externally in preparations with a maximum of 100 µg/day toxic pyrrolizidine alkaloids; commercial preparations with a very low pyrrolizidine alkaloid content are recommended

CI: Pregnancy, lactation

AE: Unknown with/for external application

I: Unknown

Comfrey Root
Symphyti radix
Symphytum officinale L.

AA: **External:** Contusions, muscle strains, bruises, and sprains; stimulation of bone healing
Local: Mouthwash and gargle with periodontis, pharyngitis, angina

D: **External/Local:** Decoction 1:10, or paste of fresh root. External preparations containing 5-20 percent of comfrey root

A: Duration of application: maximum 4 weeks/year

C: Externally in preparations with a maximum of 100 μg/day toxic pyrrolizidine alkaloids; commercial preparations with a very low pyrrolizidine alkaloid content are recommended

CI: Pregnancy, lactation

AE: Unknown for external application

I: Unknown

Common Centaury/Centaury Herb
Centaurii herba
Centaurium erythraea RAFN.

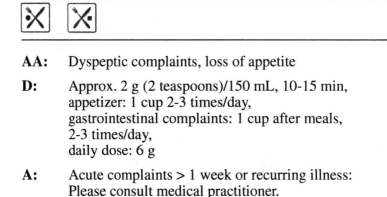

AA: Dyspeptic complaints, loss of appetite

D: Approx. 2 g (2 teaspoons)/150 mL, 10-15 min,
         appetizer: 1 cup 2-3 times/day,
         gastrointestinal complaints: 1 cup after meals,
         2-3 times/day,
         daily dose: 6 g

A: Acute complaints > 1 week or recurring illness:
         Please consult medical practitioner.

CI: Gastrointestinal ulcer

AE: Unknown

I: Unknown

Coriander
Coriandri fructus
Coriandrum sativum L.

AA: Dyspeptic complaints with mild gastrointestinal spasms, loss of appetite; feeling of fullness, flatulence

D: 1-3 g (½ teaspoon) freshly crushed/150 mL, 10-15 min, appetite enhancer → 1 cup 30 min before meals, gastrointestinal complaints → 1 cup after meals, daily dose: 3 g

A: Acute complaints > 1 week or recurring illness: Please consult medical practitioner.

CI: Unknown

AE: Unknown

I: Unknown

Corn Silk

Maidis stigma
Zea mays L.

AA: Diuretic; diseases of urinary tract

D: 0.5 g (1 teaspoon)/150 mL, cold maceration, boil and filter after a couple of minutes,
1 cup several times/day

A: Acute complaints > 1 week or recurring illness:
Please consult medical practitioner.

C: Efficacy has not been proven, no risks

CI: Unknown

AE: Unknown

I: Unknown

Couch Grass/Quack Grass
Agropyri repentis rhizoma
Agropyron repens (L.) P. BEAUV.

AA: Uriniparous for the treament of inflammatory illness of urinary tract system, prophylaxis for renal calculus and gravel; supportive therapy for catarrhs of the upper respiratory tract

D: 5-10 g (2-3 teaspoons)/150 mL, 10 min,
also cold maceration,
1 cup up to 4 times/day

A: Acute complaints > 1 week or recurring illness:
Please consult medical practitioner.

C: For cleansing/irrigation therapy: Ensure sufficient liquid intake, minimum 2 L/day. Fructose-containing additive for diabetics

CI: Not useful for dehydration or edema due to reduced heart and renal activity

AE: Unknown

I: Unknown

Cundurango/Eagle Vine
Condurango cortex
Marsdenia cundurango Reich. f.

AA: Loss of appetite, to increase gastric juice secretion, in pediatrics as aromatic bitter

D: 1.5 g (½ teaspoon)/150 mL cold water, heat to boiling point, filter after cooling down;
condurango vine: 5-10 g (3 teaspoons)/100 mL,
maceration for several days,
1 cup or liqueur glass 30 min before meals,
daily dose: 2-4 g

A: Acute complaints > 1 week or recurring illness:
Please consult medical practitioner.

CI: Unknown

AE: Unknown

I: Unknown

Damiana
Turnerae diffusae folium et herba
Turnera diffusa WILLD. ex SCHULT ssp. *gigantea*
Turnera diffusa var. *aphrodisiaca* (KINGDON-WARD) URBAN

AA: Aphrodisiac, for prophylaxis and treatment of sexual disorders; derived from Mexican traditional medicine

A: Acute complaints > 1 week or recurring illness:
Please consult medical practitioner.

C: Efficacy not proven

CI: Unknown

AE: Unknown

I: Unknown

Dandelion Root and Herb
Taraxaci radix cum herba
Taraxacum officinale WEB.

AA: Disturbance of biliary flow; dyspeptic complaints, loss of appetite; diuretic; inflammatory conditions of urinary tract

D: 3 g (2 teaspoons)/150 mL, 10 min,
1 cup 3 times/day;
tincture: 10-15 drops 3 times/day

A: Acute complaints > 1 week or recurring illness:
Please consult medical practitioner.

CI: Biliary duct blockage, bowel obstruction, and gallstones:
only with medical advice.

AE: Stomach hyperacidity

I: Unknown

Devil's Claw
Harpagophyti radix
Harpagophytum procumbens (BURCH.) DC.

AA: Dyspeptic complaints, loss of appetite; supportive therapy for degenerative complaints of locomotor system

D: Loss of appetite: 0.5-1 g (¼ teaspoon)/150 mL, 8 h,
1 cup 3 times/day before meals,
daily dose: 1.5 g
Other applications: 1.5 g (1/3 teaspoon)/150 mL, 8 h
1 cup 3 times/day,
daily dose: 4.5 g

A: Acute complaints > 1 week or recurring illness:
Please consult medical practitioner.

CI: Stomach ulcer, duodenal ulcer
Gallstones: Only with medical advice

AE: Unknown

I: Unknown

Dill
Anethi fructus
Anethum graveolens L. ssp. *graveolens*

AA: Dyspeptic disorders/diseases

D: Daily dose: 3 g (1 teaspoon)

C: Aromatic and flavor-enhancing herb

CI: Unknown

AE: Unknown

I: Unknown

Dong Quai/Danggui
Angelica sinensis radix
Angelica sinensis (OLIV.) DIELS

AA: Gynecological complaints, such as menstrual cramps, irregularities or retarded flow, weakness during the menstrual period; in TCM as a typical women's herb

D: 6-12 g/day, also in mixtures with other TCM herbs
Extract: 0.5 g/tablet or capsule, 2 tablets or capsules 2 times/day

A: Acute complaints > 1 week or recurring illness:
Please consult medical practitioner.

C: Efficacy not proven; avoid large amounts of furocoumarin-containing herbs.
Also used in cosmetic products

CI: Diarrhea, pregnancy

AE: Unknown

I: Unknown

Drosera/Sundew Herb
Drosera herba
Drosera madagascariensis DC., *D. peltata* SMITH

AA: Afflictions of respiratory tract, in particular dry cough, cough with cramp

D: 2-10 g (3-12 teaspoons)/150 mL, 10 min,
1 cup 3-4 times/day
Warning: contains naphthoquinone

A: Acute complaints > 1 week or recurring illness:
Please consult medical practitioner.

C: Naphthoquinone content varies among species: 0.006-0.6 percent → only use herbs with certified analysis

CI: Unknown

AE: Rare hypersensitivity

I: Unknown

Early Goldenrod
Solidaginis giganteaa herba
Solidago gigantea AIT. ssp. *gigantea*
[syn. S. *gigantea* AIT. var. *gigantea,*
S. *serotina* AIT. var. *gigantea* (AIT.) A. GRAY]

AA: Uriniparous effect in treatment of renal and bladder inflammation; prophylaxis and therapy of renal calculus and gravel

D: 3-5 g (2-3 teaspoons)/150 mL, 15 min,
1 cup 3-4 times/day between meals,
daily dose: 6-12 g

A: Acute complaints > 1 week or recurring illness:
Please consult medical practitioner.

C: Ensure sufficient fluid intake, minimum 2 L/day

CI: Not useful for dehydration or edema due to reduced heart and renal activity

AE: Unknown

I: Unknown

Echinacea Pallida Root
Echinaceae pallidae radix
Echinacea pallida (NUTT.) NUTT.

AA: Supportive therapy of colds and influenza

D: Daily dose: tincture 1:5 (ethanol/water 50 percent [V/V]) from native dry extract (ethanol 50 percent, monograph recommendation 7-11:1) equivalent to 900 mg herb

A: Duration of application: max 8 weeks
Acute complaints > 1 week or recurring illness:
Please consult medical practitioner.

C: Herbal teas unusual; commercial preparations containing standardized extracts are recommended.

CI: Hypersensitivity to Asteraceae;
do not use for progressive systemic diseases such as tuberculosis, leucosis, collagenosis, multiple sclerosis, and other autoimmune diseases such as HIV infection and AIDS

AE: Hypersensitivity reactions possible; exanthema, pruritus, rare facial swelling, shortness of breath, vertigo, drop in blood pressure

I: Unknown

Echinacea Purpurea Herb
Echinaceae purpureae herba
Echinacea purpurea (L.) MOENCH

AA: **Internal:** Supportive therapy for relapsing infections in respiratory tract and lower urinary tract
External: Poorly healing, superficial wounds

D: **Internal:** Daily dose: 6-9 mL pressed juice, equivalent preparations
External: Semisolid preparations, containing > 15 percent pressed juice

A: Duration of application: maximum 8 weeks
Acute complaints > 1 week or chronic illness:
Please consult medical practitioner.

C: Herbal teas unusual; commercial preparations containing standardized extracts are recommended

CI: **Internal:** Hypersensitivity to Asteraceae;
do not use for progressive systemic diseases such as tuberculosis, leucosis, collagenosis, multiple sclerosis, and other autoimmune diseases such as HIV infection and AIDS
External: Unknown

AE: Contact with aerial parts of fresh plants may cause sensitization and hypersensitive reactions; exanthema, pruritus, rare facial swelling, shortness of breath, vertigo, drop in blood pressure

I: Unknown

Eleuthero/Siberian Ginseng
Eleutherococci radix
Eleutherococcus senticosus MAXIM.

AA: Tonic for weariness, fatigue, weakness, loss of working efficiency, and decreased concentration as well as during convalescence

D: Daily dose: 2-3 g, equivalent preparations, infusions, and water-ethanolic extracts

A: Acute complaints > 1 week or recurring illness:
Please consult medical practitioner.
Duration of application: 3 months as a rule; treatment may be repeated

C: Herbal teas unusual; commercial preparations containing standardized extracts are recommended.

CI: High blood pressure

AE: Unknown

I: Unknown

English Plantain/Ribwort
Plataginis lanceolatae herba, folium
Plantago lanceolata L.

AA: **Internal:** Catarrh of respiratory tract
External: Mild inflammatory skin diseases
Local: Inflammation of mouth, throat, and pharyngeal mucosa

D: **Internal:** 1.5 g (1½ teaspoons)/150 mL, 10-15 min,
1 cup 3-4 times/day,
daily dose: 3-6 g
External/Local: 1.5 g/150 mL, cold maceration, 1-2 h,
poultice, for mouthwash and gargle

A: Acute complaints > 1 week or recurring illness:
Please consult medical practitioner.

CI: Unknown

AE: Unknown

I: Unknown

Ephedra Herb/Ma Huang
Ephedrae herba
Ephedra sinica STAPF, *E. shennungiana* TANG

AA: Diseases of the respiratory tract with mild bronchospasms such as mild forms of seasonal or chronic asthma, nasal decongestant

A: Use only with medical advice and supervision.

C: Herbal teas are dangerous and were recently banned by the FDA.
Commercial preparations containing chemically synthesized ephedrine are regulated as drugs and are recommended if medication with ephedrine is necessary.
Danger of development of tachyphylaxis and dependence
→ administration for short periods only.
Broncho dilatory efficacy of ephedrine is not always reliable.
Ephedrine-containing preparations are listed as doping agents by national and international Olympic committees.

CI: States of anxiety and restlessness, high blood pressure, angle-closure glaucoma, cerebral perfusions, prostate adenoma with residual urine volume, pheochromocytoma, thyrotoxicosis; pregnancy

AE: Sleeplessness, motor restlessness, irritability, headache, nausea, vomiting, urinary disorders, tachycardias,
higher dosages → strong rise in blood pressure and cardiac rhythm disorders

I: + cardioactive glycosides, halothane → danger of cardiac rhythm disorders;
+ monoamine oxidase inhibitors, guanethidine → potentiation of sympathomimetic effect ↑;
+ ergot alkaloids → high blood pressure ↑

Eucalyptus
Eucalypti folium
Eucalyptus globulus LABILL.

AA: Common cold, diseases of respiratory tract

D: 1.5-2 g (1 teaspoon)/150 mL, 5-10 min,
1 cup, up to 3 times/day,
daily dose: 4-6 g

A: Acute complaints > 1 week or recurring illness:
Please consult medical practitioner.

CI: Inflammatory diseases of gastrointestinal tract
and biliary ducts; severe hepatic diseases; infants < 2 y

AE: Rarely nausea, vomiting, diarrhea; allergies

I: Eucalyptus essential oil causes liver enzyme induction →
drug efficacy ↓

Eucalyptus Oil
Eucalypti aetheroleum
Eucalyptus globulus LABILL.

AA: **Internal/Inhalation:** Common cold, infections of respiratory tract
External: Common cold, infections of respiratory tract, rheumatic complaints

D: **Internal:** 3-6 drops/150 mL warm water, several times/day, daily doses: 0.3-0.6 g essential oil
External: Oily and semisolid preparations, 5-20 percent; ethanolic/water preparations, 5-10 percent;
Inhalation: 2-3 drops in hot water, vapor inhalation, single dose: 0.2 g, equivalent to 10 drops

A: Acute complaints > 1 week or recurring illness:
Please consult medical practitioner.

CI: **Internal:** Inflammatory diseases of gastrointestinal tract and bilary ducts, severe hepatic diseases
External: Babies and infants: no facial application, no inhalation
→ glottal spasms or bronchospasms could develop into asthmalike attacks and respiratory arrest

AE: Nausea, vomiting, diarrhea; allergies;
overdose → life-threatening intoxication;
children (a few drops), adults (> 4-5 mL)
→ blood pressure ↓, collapse, respiratory paralysis

I: Liver enzyme induction → drug efficacy ↓

European Goldenrod
Solidaginis virgaureae herba
Solidago virgaurea L.

AA: To increase urine volume with inflammatory diseases of the urinary tract; therapy and prophylaxis with renal calculus and gravel

D: 3-5 g (2-3 teaspoons)/150 mL, 15 min,
1 cup between meals 2-4 times/day,
daily dose: 6-12 g

A: Acute complaints > 1 week or recurring illness:
Please consult medical practitioner.

C: Ensure suffucient fluid intake, minimum 2 L/day

CI: Not useful for dehydration or edema due to reduced heart and renal activity

AE: Unknown

I: Unknown

European Mistletoe
Visci (albi) herba
Viscum album L.

AA: **Internal:** As adjuvant for the treatment of cases of mild high blood pressure, vertigo
Parenteral: Nonspecific stimulation for treating degenerative inflammation of the joints, when strong local inflammatory effect is desired
As palliative therapy for malignant tumors as a nonspecific irritatant

D: **Internal:** 2.5 g (1 teaspoon)/150 mL cold water, 10-12 h, before drinking heat to boiling point, 1-2 cups/day
Parenteral: According to package insert in commercial preparations

A: Use only with medical advice and supervision.
Efficacy of parenteral administration does not necessarily apply to herbal tea.

C: Efficacy in the treatment of cases of mild high blood pressure (borderline hypertonia) not sufficiently documented.

CI: Parenteral administration: Protein oversensitivity, chronic progressive infections, as, for example, tuberculosis, high fever

AE: Parenteral administration: Local reactions could occur (welt formation, possibly also necroses), chills, fever, headache, anginal complaints, orthostatic circulatory disorders, and allergic reactions

I: Unknown

Eyebright Herb
Euphrasiae herba
Euprasia stricta WOLFF ex. J. F. LEHM.

⊘

AA: **External:** For eye complaints associated with disorders and inflammation of the blood vessels, inflammation of the eye-lids and conjunctiva; as lotions, poultices, and eye baths

D: Infusion: 2-3 g (1-2 teaspoons)/150 mL, 5-10 min,
decoction: 3 g/150 mL, 5-10 min,
3-4 times/day for eye rinse

A: Acute complaints > 1 week or recurring illness:
Please consult medical practioner.

C: Efficacy is not proven, application not recommended for hygienic reasons;
filtered, sterile extracts may be applied using an eyecup.

CI: *See* C

AE: Unknown

I: Unknown

Fennel

Foeniculi fructus
Foeniculum vulgare MILL., var. *vulgare,* var. *dulce*

AA: Dyspeptic conditions such as mild gastrointestinal cramps, feeling of fullness or repletion as well as tympanites; catarrh of the respiratory tract

D: 2.5 g (1 teaspoon) freshly crushed/150 mL, 10-15 min covered,
1 cup 2-3 times/day,
daily dose: 5-7 g

A: Acute complaints > 1 week or recurring illness:
Please consult medical practitioner.

C: Sweet and bitter varieties of the herb, the latter applied medicinally

CI: Preparations containing amounts of volatile components comparable to infusions: unknown

AE: Individual cases of allergic reactions of skin and airways

I: Unknown

Fenugreek Seed
Foenugraeci semen
Trigonella foenum-graecum L.

AA: **Internal:** Loss of appetite
External: Local inflammation

D: **Internal:** 2 g crushed drug taken with fluid 3 times/day before meals;
cold maceration: 0.5 g (¼ teaspoon)/150 mL, 3 h, 1 cup several times/day,
daily dose: 6 g
External: Poultice: boil 50 g powdered seeds with 250 mL, 5 min, once/day

A: Acute complaints > 1 week or recurring illness:
Please consult medical practitioner.

CI: Pregnancy

AE: Sensitization is possible through repeated external administration of the herb.

I: Unknown

Feverfew Herb
Tanaceti parthenii herba
Tanacetum parthenium (L.) SCHULTZ BIP.

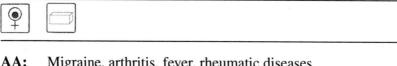

AA: Migraine, arthritis, fever, rheumatic diseases

D: Powdered herb: daily dose 50-1,200 mg

A: Acute complaints > 1 week or recurring illness:
          Please consult medical practitioner.

C: Herbal teas unusual; commercial preparations containing
          standardized extracts are recommended.

CI: Pregnancy, lactation; hypersensitivity to Asteraceae

AE: Ulceration of mouth mucosa, abdominal pain, digestive dis-
          orders; overdose → vertigo, cramps, shortness of breath,
          coma

I: Unknown

Frangula Bark/Buckthorn Bark
Frangulae cortex
Rhamnus frangula L.

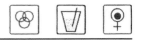

AA: Constipation

D: Up to 2 g (½ teaspoon)/150 mL, 10-15 min,
1 cup freshly brewed in the morning and/or in the evening,
daily dose: 20-30 mg hydroxyanthraquinone derivatives
The individual correct dosage is the lowest that is necessary
to obtain a smooth stool.

A: Duration of application: short-term therapy (maximum 1-2
weeks).
Please consult medical practitioner.

C: Long-term application may cause intensification of digestive
disorder. Nutrition may be enriched by vegetable fibers;
ensure sufficient fluid intake and body movement.

CI: Intestinal blockage; acute inflammatory intestinal illness
(Crohn's disease, ulcerative colitis, appendicitis); abdominal
pains of unknown cause;
children < 12 y; pregnancy and lactation

AE: Individual cases of gastrointestinal cramping;
frequent and long-term application or overdose may lead to
loss of electrolytes (potassium), albuminuria, hematuria

I: Deprivation of potassium → effect of cardioactive glycosides
↑; influences the effect of antiarrhythmics

Fucus/Kelp
Fucus vesiculosus
Fucus vesiculosus L.

AA: Disease of thyroid gland, adiposity, overweight, arteriosclerosis, disgestive disorders, as well as "blood purifying"

C: Efficacy not proven; therapeutic application not recommended

Note: Contains iodine salts

> 150 μg iodine/day → induction and deterioration of hyperthyroidism possible

AE: Rare cases of severe reactions of hypersensitivity

Fumitory Herb/Earth Smoke
Fumariae herba
Fumaria officinalis L.

$\boxed{\times}$

AA: Cramps as well as gastrointestinal disturbances of gallbladder and biliary ducts

D: 2-4 g (1-2 teaspoons)/150 mL, 10 min,
1 cup, warm, 2-3 times/day 30 min before meals,
daily dose: 6 g

A: Acute complaints > 1 week or recurring illness:
Please consult medical practitioner.

CI: Unknown

AE: Unknown

I: Unknown

Galangal/Chinese Ginger/Galanga
Galangae rhizoma
Alpinia officinarum HANCE

☒

AA: Loss of appetite, dyspeptic complaints

D: 0.5-1 g (1/3 teaspoon)/150 mL, 5-10 min covered,
1 cup 30 min before meals,
daily dose: 2-4 g

A: Acute complaints > 1 week or recurring illness:
Please consult medical practitioner.

CI: Unknown

AE: Unknown

I: Unknown

Garlic/Garlic Oil
Allii sativi bulbus, oleum
Allium sativum L.

AA: Adjuvant to dietetic measures for raised blood lipid levels; preventive measures for age-related vascular changes and arteriosclerosis, effects concentration-dependent

D: Average daily dose: 4 g fresh garlic or 8 mg oil, commercial preparations accordingly

A: Acute complaints > 1 week or recurring illness:
Please consult medical practitioner.

C: Used as sap/juice, distillate, garlic oil maceration, powder; fresh bulbs as spice; preparations phytochemically different. Infusions/decoctions ineffective. Bad breath and skin odor depending on concentration.

CI: Lactation

AE: Rare cases of gastrointestinal complaints and allergic reactions (hand eczema)

I: Unknown

Gentian

Gentianae radix
Gentiana lutea L.

☒

AA: Digestive complaints due to reduced gastric juice secretion; loss of appetite, feeling of fullness, bloating, and flatulence

D: 1 g (1/3 teaspoon)/150 mL, 10-15 min,
1 cup several times/day
appetite enhancer → 30 min before meals,
digestive disorders → after meals,
drink cold or tepid,
daily dose: 2-4 g

A: Acute complaints > 1 week or recurring illness:
Please consult medical practitioner.

C: Component of Swedish bitters

CI: Gastric and duodenal ulcers

AE: Rare cases of headache for sensitive persons

I: Unknown

Ginger/Ginger Root
Zingiberis rhizoma
Zingiber officinalis ROSC.

AA: Dyspeptic complaints, motion sickness; appetite enhancer

D: Dyspeptic complaints: 0.5-1.0 g (1/3 teaspoon)/150 mL, 1 cup 2-4 times/day
Tincture: 3 × 20 drops/day
Antiemetic: 2 g (1 scant teaspoon) freshly powdered herb taken with some liquid,
daily dose: 2-4 g

A: Acute complaints > 1 week or recurring illness:
Please consult medical practitioner.

C: Motion sickness: 250 mg powered herb in commercial preparations

CI: Vomiting during pregnancy, morning sickness; gallstones: Only with medical advice

AE: Unknown

I: Unknown

Ginkgo/Ginkgo Biloba Extract
Ginkgo bilobae folium, extractum siccatum
Ginkgo biloba L.

AA: Symptomatic therapy of disturbed brain functions; peripheral arterial occlusive diseases (Stage II according to Fontaine); vertigo, tinnitus; antidementive

D: According to package insert in commercial preparations

C: Efficacy proven for special extracts; not proven for herbal tea preparations.
Herbal teas unusual; commercial preparations containing standardized extracts are recommended.

CI: Hypersensitivity to *ginkgo biloba* preparations

AE: Very rare cases of gastrointestinal complaints, headache, allergic skin reactions

I: Unknown

Goldenseal/Hydrastis
Hydrastis rhizoma
Hydrastis canadensis L.

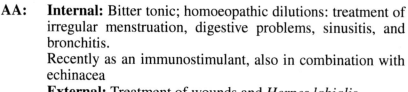

AA: **Internal:** Bitter tonic; homoeopathic dilutions: treatment of irregular menstruation, digestive problems, sinusitis, and bronchitis.
Recently as an immunostimulant, also in combination with echinacea
External: Treatment of wounds and *Herpes labialis*

D: **Internal:** 0.5-1.0 g (2 teaspoons)/150 mL, 10 min,
1 cup 3 times/day
External: fluid extract 0.2-1.0 mL

A: Acute complaints > 1 week or recurring illness:
Please consult medical practitioner.

C: Efficacy not yet proven; therapeutic application not recommended

CI: Pregnancy, lactation

AE: Long-term therapy → digestive disorders, constipation, excitatory states, hallucinations, and occasionally delirium.
High doses → vomiting, difficulty in breathing, bradycardia, spasms, eventually leading to central paralysis

I: Long-term use: reduction of vitamin B absorption possible

Grape Seed
Vitis semen
Vitis vinifera L.

AA: Antioxidant, scavenger of free radicals, inhibitor of lipid peroxidation

D: Daily dose: 50 mg for general health purposes

A: Acute complaints > 1 week or recurring illness:
Please consult medical practitioner.

C: Commercial preparations standardized on the basis of procyanidin content

CI: Unknown

AE: Unknown

I: Unknown

Great Burnet Saxifrage/Saxifrage
Pimpinellae radix
Pimpinella major (L.) HUDS., *P. saxifraga* L.

AA: Catarrh of the upper respiratory tract

D: 2-4 g (1-2 teaspoons)/150 mL,
1 cup up to 3 times/day,
daily dose: 6-12 g respectively 6-15 mL tincture (1:5)

A: Acute complaints > 1 week or recurring illness:
Please consult medical practitioner.

CI: Unknown

AE: Photosensitization possible, particularly for persons with light skin

I: Unknown

Greater Celandine
Chelidonii herba
Chelidonium majus L.

☒	⚲

AA: Cramplike gastrointestinal disturbances, biliary duct complaints

D: 0.5-1 g (½-1 teaspoon)/150 mL, 10 min,
1 cup 3 times/day between meals;
daily dose: 2-5 mg respectively 12-30 mg total alkaloids, calculated as chelidonine

A: Acute complaints > 1 week or recurring illness:
Please consult medical practitioner.

C: Commercial preparations containing standardized extracts are recommended. Herbal teas are not recommended.

CI: Pregnancy

AE: Unknown

I: Unknown

Greek Sage Leaf
Salviae trilobae folium
Salvia triloba L. FIL.

AA: Inflammation of mouth, throat, and pharyngeal mucosa; gingivitis, sore gums due to wearing dentures

D: 3 g (3-4 teaspoons)/150 mL, 10 min,
warm decoction used for gargle and cleansing, several times/ day

A: Acute complaints > 1 week or recurring illness:
Please consult medical practitioner.

C: Unknown

CI: Unknown

AE: Unknown

I: Unknown

Guggul/Guggal
Bdellium indicum
Commiphora mukul (HOOK. ex. STOCKS) ENGL.

AA: In traditional Indian medicine for rheumatic fever; effect in lowering serum cholesterol and triglyceride levels

A: Acute complaints > 1 week or recurring illness:
Please consult medical practitioner.

C: Efficacy not yet sufficiently proven. The powdered resin is available in the form of capsules in the United States.

CI: Unknown

AE: Unknown

I: Unknown

Haronga/Harungana Bark, Leaf
Harunganae madagascariensis cortex et folium
Harungana madagascariensis LAM. ex POIR.

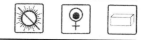

AA: Dyspeptic complaints and mild pancreatic insufficiency

D: Daily dose: 7.5-15 mg of dry extract (ethanol/water) equivalent to 25-50 mg herb, 3-4 single doses

A: Acute complaints > 1 week or recurring illness: Please consult medical practitioner. Do not apply > 2 months

C: Herbal teas unusual; commercial preparations containing standardized extracts are recommended.

CI: Acute pancreatitis, acute episode of chronic pancreatitis, severe liver function disorders, gallstone illnesses, obstruction of the biliary ducts, gallbladder empyema or ileus. Children < 12 y; pregnancy and lactation

AE: Photosensitization is possible particularly for persons with light/fair skin, but unlikely due to low therapeutic dosage.

I: Unknown

Hawthorn Herb with Flower/Haw/White Thorn
Crataegi folium cum flore
Crataegus monogyna JAQC.

AA:　Mild cardiac insufficiency (Stage II NYHA), geriatric heart illnesses

D:　1-1.5 g (1 teaspoon)/150 mL, 5-10 min,
1 cup 3-4 times/day,
daily dose: 5 g
3.5-19.8 mg flavonoids or 160-900 mg extract
(4-7:1 ethanol 45 percent V/V or methanol 70 percent V/V)
equivalent to 30-168.7 mg oligomeric procyanidines, calculated as epicatechin, or 3.5-19.8 mg flavonoids calculated as hyperoside

A:　Duration of treatment: minimum 6 weeks
Symptoms > 6 weeks or edema in the legs:
Please consult medical practitioner.
Pain in cardiac region, shortness of breath, respiratory distress: Consult medical practitioner immediately.

C:　Commercial preparations containing standardized extracts are recommended; efficacy of the fruits (Crataegi fructus) not proven

CI:　Unknown

AE:　Unknown

I:　Unknown

Hayseed flower
Graminis flos
Graminaceae, meadow flowers

AA: Local heat treatment for degenerative diseases of rheumatic origin

D: Bag filled with hayseed covered with boiling water,
5 min,
externally as hot moist compress,
approx. 42°C, 30-60 min

A: Use bag only once for hygenic reasons

C: Consisting of grasses and meadow flowers 1:1

CI: Open injuries; acute, rheumatic phase; acute inflammation; allergy to grass pollen

AE: Rare allergic skin reactions possible

I: Unknown

Heartsease/Wild Pansy
Violae tricoloris herba
Viola tricolor L.

AA: Mild seborrheic skin diseases;
         milk crust, cradle cap in children

D: 1.5 g (1 teaspoon)/150 mL, 10 min,
         hip bath, poultice, several times/day

A: Acute complaints > 1 week or recurring illness:
         Please consult medical practitioner.

CI: Unknown

AE: Unknown

I: Unknown

Hemp Nettle
Galeopsidis herba
Galeopsis segetum NECKER

AA: Mild coughs and bronchitis, catarrh of airways; pediatrics

D: 2 g (2 teaspoons)/150 mL, 5 min,
also cold maceration, heat for 5 min,
1 cup several times/day,
average daily dose: 6 g

A: Acute complaints > 1 week or recurring illness:
Please consult medical practitioner.

CI: Unknown

AE: Unknown

I: Unknown

Henna
Hennae folium
Lawsonia inermis L.

AA: Hair, skin, and nail coloring agent

D: Powdered leaves mixed with hot water → pulp.
Intensity of coloring effect dependent on application time:
the longer, the stronger.
Test duration of application on single strand of hair.
Adding lemon juice or red wine →
As effect of tannins ↑ → brown colors ↑

A: After applying the pulp, the head should be covered.

C: Brownish hair + henna → reddish
light blond + henna → carrot-red
chestnut brown + henna → mahogany red
henna neutral, noncoloring → shiny hair

AE: Skin sensitization, contact dermatitis; frequent application →
delayed hypersensitivity reactions possible, individual cases
of immediate reactions reported

I: Unknown

Herniary/Rupturewort
Herniariae herba
Herniaria glabra L.

○

AA: Renal disorders and complaints of derivative urinary tract, respiratory tract complaints

D: 1.5 g (1 teaspoon)/150 mL, cold maceration, boil for 5 min, as diuretic 1 cup 2-3 times/day

A: Acute complaints > 1 week or recurring illness: Please consult medical practitioner.

C: Efficacy not yet proven; no risks

CI: Unknown

AE: Unknown

I: Unknown

Hibiscus Flower/Jamaica Sorrel/Roselle
Hibisci flos
Hibiscus sabdariffa L.

AA: Loss of appetite, common cold, catarrh of upper respiratory tract and stomach; higher amounts → mild laxative; mainly used as aromatic and flavor-enhancing herb, ornamental herb

D: 1.5 g (½ teaspoon)/150 mL, 5-10 min,
1 cup 5-10 times/day

A: Acute complaints > 1 week or recurring illness:
Please consult medical practitioner.

C: Efficacy not proven; no risks; safe when used as ornamental herb and as indicated

CI: Unknown

AE: Unknown

I: Unknown

Hops
Lupuli strobulus
Humulus lupulus L.

AA: Restlessness and anxiety; initial insomnia

D: 0.5 g (1-2 teaspoons)/150 mL, 10-15 min,
1 cup 2-3 times/day
and 1 cup before going to sleep,
single dose: 0.5 g,
as sedative: single dose: 1-2 g

A: Acute complaints > 1 week or recurring illness:
Please consult medical practitioner.

C: Combination with other sedative herbs permissible (different dosage)

CI: Unknown

AE: Unknown

I: Unknown

Horehound/Hoarhound

Marrubii herba
Marrubium vulgare L.

[⊕♀]

AA: Dyspeptic conditions such as feeling of fullness, bloating, and flatulence, loss of appetite, catarrh of the respiratory tract

D: 1.5 g (1-2 teaspoons)/150 mL, 10 min,
1 cup 3 times/day,
daily dose: 4.5 g
Pressed juice: 2-6 tablespoons/day
Fluid extract (1:1): 2-4 mL, 3 times/day

A: Acute complaints > 1 week or recurring illness:
Please consult medical practitioner.

CI: Pregnancy

AE: Unknown when used as indicated

I: Unknown

Horny Goat Weed/Barrenwort

Epimedium spp.
Several species as botanical sources (*E. acuminatum,*
E. brevicornum, E. davidii, E. hunanense,
E. koreanum, E. pubescens, E. sagittarum,
E. wushanense)

AA: Used in TCM as a tonic and in the treatment of rheumatic and paralytic diseases and involutional hypertension; regulation of immunulogical functions

D: Isolated natural products from *Epimedium* spp. and extracts of different polarities are applied in TCM

A: Acute complaints > 1 week or recurring illness:
Please consult medical practitioner.

C: The clinical applications of *Epimedium* in TCM are numerous. A medical practitioner experienced in TCM should be consulted.

Horse Chestnut Seed
Hippocastani semen
Aesculus hippocastanum L.

AA: **Internal:** Complaints of leg veins (CVI) for such symptoms as pain and heaviness of the legs, nocturnal calf cramps, itchiness, and swelling of the legs
External: Traumatic swelling such as sports injuries and bruising; hemorrhoids, CVI

D: **Internal:** Daily dose: 100 mg aescin (1 mg aescin/kg body weight), equivalent to 250-312.5 mg extract in delayed-action/slow-release commercial herb preparations
External: In ointments at different concentrations, apply 1-2 times/day

A: Acute complaints > 1 week or recurring illness:
Please consult medical practitioner.

C: Additional actions such as compression bandages/stockings and cold effusions should be taken by all means. Herbal teas unusual; commercial preparations containing standardized extracts are recommended.

CI: Unknown

AE: Individual cases of itching, nausea, indigestion

I: Unknown

Horsetail
Equiseti herba
Equisetum arvense L.

AA: **Internal:** Cleansing therapy with bacterial and inflammatory illness of derivative urinary tract, with gravel; posttraumatic and static edema;
External: Supportive therapy to promote wound healing

D: **Internal:** 2-3 g (2-3 teaspoons)/150 mL, 10-15 min, 1 cup 3 times/day, daily dose: 6 g
External: Compresses: 10 g drug to 1 L

A: Acute complaints > 1 week or recurring illness: Please consult medical practitioner.

C: Ensure sufficient fluid intake, minimum 2 L/day.

CI: Not useful for dehydration or edema due to reduced heart and renal activity

AE: Unknown

I: Unknown

Iceland Moss
Lichen islandicus
Cetraria islandica (L.) ACH.

AA: **Internal:** Expectorant for dry cough; loss of appetite
        Local: Irritation of mouth, throat, and pharyngeal mucosa

D: **Internal:** 1.5 g (1 teaspoon)/150 mL, 10-15 min,
        1 cup 3-4 times/day;
        as appetite enhancer before meals: 1 cup 3-4 times/day,
        cold maceration: 1.5 g (1 teaspoon)/150 mL,
        1-2 h cold, heat to boiling point
        Local: Gargle and cleansing, prepare accordingly

A: Acute complaints > 1 week or recurring illness:
        Please consult medical practitioner.

C: Immune-stimulating effects not yet proven

CI: Unknown

AE: **Local:** Individual cases of sensitization

I: Unknown

Indian Frankincense
Olibanum
Boswellia carteri BIRDW.

Indian Olibanum Tree
Olibanum
Boswellia serrata ROXB. EX COLEBR.

AA: Chronic inflammatory intestinal illnesses (colitis ulcerosa, Chron's disease), bronchial asthma; in traditional Indian medicine, treatment of chronic rheumatic inflammation

D: Standardized dry extract recommended

A: Acute complaints > 1 week or recurring illness:
Please consult medical practitioner.

C: Efficacy is not yet proven.

Frankincense or olibanum is the gum resin of the trunk of *Boswellia carteri* (Birdw.), exuded when incisions are made in the trunk, and hardened in the open air.
Indian frankincense or olibanum is the gum resin of the trunk of *Boswellia serrata* (Roxb. ex Colebr.), exuded when incisions are made in the trunk, and hardened in the open air.

CI: Unknown

AE: Unknown when used as indicated in package insert or with indicated usage

I: Unknown

Ipecacuanha Root/Ipecac
Ipecacuanhae radix
Psychotria ipecacuanha (BROT.) STOKES

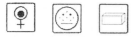

AA: Amebic dysentery, expectorant for chronic bronchitis, initial treatment for acute bronchitis; higher dosage: as an emetic in cases of poisoning, treatment of bronchitis with croupy cough in children

D: Infusion: 0.5 g/100 mL
single dose: 10 mL (adults);
emetic effect: single dose: 0.5-2 g
tincture: 0.5 g (approx. 27 drops) with some liquid

A: Use only with medical advice and supervision.

C: Herbal teas not advised due to risk of overdose; commercial preparations containing standardized extracts are recommended.

CI: Pregnancy

AE: Generally, skin and mucosa irritation; frequent contact with the herb → allergic reactions of the skin and the mucous membranes ("druggist's asthma"; the allergen is a glyco-protein); long time administration → myopathies

I: Unknown

Ivy/English Ivy
Hederae helicis folium
Hedera helix L.

AA: Symptomatic treatment of chronic inflammatory bronchial conditions (adjuvant); catarrhs of the respiratory tract such as pertussis and spastic bronchitis

D: Average daily dose: 0.3 g (1/3 teaspoon; 1 teaspoon equivalent to 1 g)

A: Acute complaints > 1 week or recurring illness: Please consult medical practitioner.

C: Herbal teas unusual due to low average daily dose; commercial preparations containing standardized extracts are recommended.

CI: Known allergies to ivy and ivy preparations

AE: Sensitization possible

I: Unknown

Java Citronella Oil
Citronellae aetheroleum
Cymbopogon winterianus IOWITT.

AA: Treatment of mild unrest and nervous conditions (no organic causes)

D: ¾ bath: at least 4.0 g essential oil/100 L

A: Acute complaints > 1 week or recurring illness:
Please consult medical practitioner.

C: Ingredient in cosmetic preparations; insect repellent

CI: Skin injuries, skin diseases, severe febrile infectious diseases; heart insufficiency, hypertonia

AE: Unknown

I: Unknown

Java Tea
Orthosiphonis folium
Orthosiphon aristatus (BLUME) MIQ.

AA: Cleansing therapy with bacterial and inflammatory illness of derivative urinary tract, irritable bladder, and gravel

D: 2 g (1 teaspoon)/150 mL, 10-15 min,
1 cup several times/day,
daily dose: 6-12 g

A: Acute complaints > 1 week or recurring illness:
Please consult medical practitioner.

C: Ensure sufficient fluid intake, minimum 2 L/day

CI: Not useful for dehydration or edema due to reduced heart and renal activity

AE: Unknown

I: Unknown

Juniper Berry
Juniperi fructus
Juniperus communis L.

AA: **Internal:** Digestive complaints with mild cramps, feeling of fullness, and flatulence
External: Bath additive of supportive therapy for rheumatic diseases

D: **Internal:** 2 g (1 scant teaspoon), freshly ground/150 mL, 10-15 min,
1 cup 1-4 times/day,
daily dose: 2 g to maximum 10 g, equivalent to 20-100 mg volatile oil

A: Acute complaints > 1 week or recurring illness:
Please consult medical practitioner.
Duration of treatment: maximum 6 weeks

C: Combination with other diuretic herbs ("bladder-and-kidney tea") may be useful

CI: Pregnancy, inflammatory renal diseases; no local application with extensive skin lesions; therapeutic full baths with feverish and infectious diseases, cardiac insufficiency Stage III-IV (NYHA), hypertonia Stage IV (WHO): only after consulting medical practitioner

AE: Long-term internal application or overdose: kidney irritation and damage possible

I: Unknown

Khella/Visnaga
Ammeos visnagae fructus
Ammi visnaga (L.) LAM.

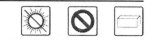

AA: Angina pectoris, cardiac insufficiency, paroxysmal tachycardia, extra systoles, presbycardia with hypertonia, asthma, pertussis, and abdominal cramps

C: Efficacy not proven; therapeutic application of the herb not advised; commercial preparations containing standardized extracts are recommended.

AE: Long-term use or overdose of the herb: nausea, dizziness, loss of appetite, headache, sleep disorders possible; cases of very high doses (corresponding to over 100 mg khellin): elevated levels (reversible) of liver enzymes in blood plasma; infrequently, a cholestatic jaundice (reversible); phototoxic effect

Lady's Mantle/Lion's Foot
Alchemilae herba
Alchemilla xanthochlora ROTHM.

☒

AA: Mild, nonspecific diarrhea

D: 2 g (2 teaspoons)/150 mL, 10-15 min,
1 cup between meals 3-5 times/day;
daily dose: 5-10 g

A: For diarrhea > 3-4 days: Please consult medical practitioner.

CI: Do not use for diarrhea in babies and infants. Consult pediatrician in all cases

AE: Unknown

I: Unknown

Lavender Flower
Lavandulae flos
Lavandula angustifolia MILL.

AA: **Internal:** Restlessness, initial insomnia, loss of appetite, functional abdominal complaints, nervous stomach irritation, tympanites, nervous intestinal complaints
External: Balneotherapy for treatment of functional circulatory disorders

D: **Internal:** 1-1.5 g (1-2 teaspoons)/150 mL,
10 min covered,
3 cups/day, especially before going to sleep
External: 100-500 g/100 L water

A: Acute complaints > 1 week or recurring illness:
Please consult medical practitioner.

C: Combination with other sedative herbs may be useful.

CI: Unknown; no local application with extensive skin lesions; therapeutic full baths with feverish and infectious diseases, cardiac insufficiency Stage III-IV (NYHA), hypertonia Stage IV (WHO): only after consulting medical practitioner

AE: Unknown

I: Unknown

Lavender Oil
Lavandulae aetheroleum
Lavandula angustifolia MILL.

AA: Restlessness, initial insomnia, loss of appetite, functional abdominal complaints, nervous stomach irritation, tympanites, nervous intestinal complaints

D: 1-4 drops (approx. 20-80 mg) on a piece of sugar

A: Acute complaints > 1 week or recurring illness:
Please consult medical practitioner.

C: Combination with other sedative and/or carminative herbs may be useful

CI: Unknown

AE: Unknown; individual cases of allergies

I: Unknown

Licorice Root/Glycyrrhiza
Liquiritiae radix
Glycyrrhiza glabra L.

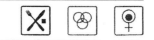

AA: Catarrh of the upper respiratory tract, gastric duodenal ulcers, chronic gastritis

D: 4-5 g (1-2 teaspoons)/150 mL, 10-15 min,
1 cup 2-3 times/day after meals,
daily dose: herb: 5-15 g, equivalent to 200-600 mg glycyrrhizin
licorice sap: 0.5-1 g for catarrh of the upper respiratory tract, 1.5-3 g for gastric and duodenal ulcer

A: With high doses, not longer than 6 weeks without medical advice

CI: Chronic hepatitis, cholestatic diseases of the liver, cirrhosis of the liver, severe renal insufficiency, hypertonia, hypokalemia; pregnancy

AE: Higher doses (above 50 g/day) and/or long-term therapy → potassium ↓, natrium ↑, edemas, hypertension and cardiac complaints, in rare cases myoglobinemia

I: + thiazide/loop diuretic → deprivation of potassium;
→ raised cardiac glycosides

Linden Flower/Lime Tree Flower
Tiliae flos
Tilia cordata MILL., *T. platyphyllos* SCOP., *T. vulgaris* HEYNE

AA: Catarrh of the respiratory tract, irritable dry cough; as a diaphoretic for colds with fever and for infectious diseases

D: 2 g (1 teaspoon)/150 mL, 5-10 min,
also cold maceration, heat to boiling point, 5-10 min, 1-2 times/day
daily dose: 2-4 g

A: Acute complaints > 1 week or recurring illness:
Please consult medical practitioner.

CI: Unknown

AE: Unknown

I: Unknown

Linseed/Flaxseed
Lini semen
Linum usitatissimum L.

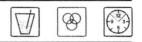

AA: **Internal:** Chronic constipation, irritable colon, diverticulitis, gastritis, and enteritis
External: Poultice for local skin infections

D: **Internal:** Approx. 10 g (2 teaspoons) of whole or bruised (not ground) seed with at least 150 mL of liquid
2 times/day
Linseed gruel for gastritis, enteritis: approx. 10 g (2 teaspoons)/150 mL of milled linseed
External: 30-50 g linseed meal for a hot moist poultice

A: Acute complaints > 1 week or recurring illness:
Please consult medical practitioner.

C: Ensure sufficient fluid intake, minimum 2 L/day.

CI: Intestinal blockage; narrowed esophagus or entrance to the stomach, acute inflammatory intestinal illness (Crohn's disease, ulcerative colitis, appendicitis);
children < 6 y

AE: Unknown

I: The absorption of other medication administered concomitantly may be inhibited (e.g., iron-lithium preparations from gastrointestinal tract) → 30 min interval after administration

Lovage Root
Levistici radix
Levisticum officinale KOCH

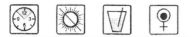

AA: Cleansing therapy with bacterial and inflammatory illness of derivative urinary tract, as a prophylaxis for kidney gravel; also for dyspeptic complaints such as indigestion, heartburn, feelings of fullness, flatulence

D: 2-4 g (1 teaspoon)/150 mL, 10-15 min,
1 cup several times/day between meals;
stomachic: 1 cup 30 min before meals
daily dose; 4-8 g

A: Acute complaints > 1 week or recurring illness:
Please consult medical practitioner.

C: Ensure sufficient fluid intake, minimum 2 L/day.

CI: Inflammatory diseases of the kidneys or urinary drainage passages, reduced cardiac and renal function; pregnancy

AE: Individual cases of photodermatosis; long-term therapy →
avoid exposure to direct sunlight or intensive UV radiation

I: Unknown

Lycopodium/Club Moss
Lycopodii herba
Lycopodium clavatum L.

AA: Bladder and renal complaints; diuretic

D: 1.5 g (1-2 teaspoons)/150 mL, 10-15 min,
1 cup 2-3 times/day

A: Acute complaints > 1 week or recurring illness:
Please consult medical practitioner.

C: Efficacy not proven

CI: Unknown

AE: Long-term use may cause mucosa irritation.

I: Unknown

Mallow Leaf and Flower

Malvae folium, Malvae flos
Malva neglecta WALLR., *Malva sylvestris* ssp. *mauritiana* (L.)
BOISS. ex COUT

AA: Irritations of mouth, throat, and pharyngeal mucosa as well as the gastrointestinal tract, catarrh of the upper respiratory tract, and dry irritable cough; mild astringent for gastro-enteritis

D: 3-5 g leaves (3-4 teaspoons)/150 mL, 10 min,
1.5-2 g flowers (3-4 teaspoons)/150 mL, 10 min,
also cold maceration, 1 cup several times/day,
daily dose: 3-5 g

A: Acute complaints > 1 week or recurring illness:
Please consult medical practitioner.

C: Mallow flowers are also used as ornamental herb.

CI: Unknown

AE: Unknown

I: Unknown

Manna
Manna cannelata
Fraxinus ornus L.

AA: Ailments for which an easier elimination and a smooth stool is desirable, such as anal fissures, hemorrhoids, and constipation; preoperative medication

D: Adults, daily dose: 20-30 g
children, daily dose: 2-16 g
1 teaspoon equivalent to 3-4 g

A: Acute complaints > 1 week or recurring illness:
Please consult medical practitioner.

C: Component of Swedish bitters

CI: Intestinal occlusion

AE: Flatulence and nausea possible

I: Unknown

Marshmallow Leaf
Althaeae folium
Althaea officinalis L.

AA: **Internal:** Soothing of irritable cough
Local: Inflammations of mouth, throat, and pharyngeal mucosa

D: **Internal:** 1-2 g (2 teaspoons)/150 mL, 10 min,
also cold maceration, 1 h,
1 cup, slightly tepid, several times/day,
daily dose: 5 g
Local: Gargle and cleansing; for dosage *see* INTERNAL

A: Acute complaints > 1 week or recurring illness:
Please consult medical practitioner.

CI: Unknown

AE: Unknown

I: The absorption of other medication administered concomitantly may be retarded.

Marshmallow Root
Althaeae radix
Althaea officinalis L.

AA: **Internal:** Soothing of irritable cough, mild inflammation of gastric mucosa
Local: Inflammations of mouth, throat, and pharyngeal mucosa
External: Inflammations, ulcers, abscesses of the skin, and skin burns

D: **Internal:** 2 g (1/2 teaspoon)/150 mL cold water, stir frequently for 90 min, heat to boiling point, 1 cup, slightly tepid, several times/day, daily dose: 6 g
External: Poultice with aqueous extracts

A: Acute complaints > 1 week or recurring illness: Please consult medical practitioner.

CI: Unknown

AE: Unknown

I: The absorption of other medication administered concomitantly may be retarded.

Maté/Paraguay Tea
Mate folium
Ilex paraguariensis ST.-HIL.

AA: Mental and physical fatigue

D: Approx. 2 g (1 teaspoon)/150 mL, 5-10 min;
steeped for a shorter period of time → more stimulating, less
astringent, more pleasant taste;
caffeine dissolves faster than tannins;
daily dose: 3 g

A: Acute complaints > 1 week or recurring illness:
Please consult medical practitioner.

CI: Unknown

AE: Unknown

I: Unknown

Meadowsweet Flower and Herb
Filipendula ulmariae flos, F. ulmariae herba
Filipendula ulmaria var. *vulgare* (L.) MAXIM.

AA: Supportive therapy for colds (flowers and herb); for febrile colds as a diuretic (flowers)

D: 1-2 g (1 teaspoon)/150 mL, 10 min,
1 cup several times/day as hot as possible,
daily dose: flower, 2.5-3.5 g; herb, 4-5 g

A: Acute complaints > 1 week or recurring illness:
Please consult medical practitioner.

C: Flower therapeutically more valuable

CI: Known allergy or hypersensitivity to salicylate due to salicylate content

AE: Unknown

I: Unknown

Melilot/King's Clover
Meliloti herba
Melilotus officinalis (L.) PALL., *M. altissima* THUILL.

AA: **Internal:** Symptoms of CVI complaints such as heavy and painful legs, nocturnal calf pain (night cramps in the legs), pruritus, and swelling;
supportive therapy for thrombophlebitis, postthrombotic syndromes, hemorrhoidal complaints, and lymphatic congestion
External: Contusions, sprains, and superficial bruises

D: **Internal:** 1.5-3 g (1 teaspoon)/150 mL, 5-10 min,
1 cup 2-3 times/day,
daily dose: herb or preparations equivalent to 3-30 mg coumarin
External: Poultice for hemorrhoids,
for dosage, *see* INTERNAL

A: Acute complaints > 1 week or recurring illness:
Please consult medical practitioner.

CI: Unknown

AE: Very high doses → headache and stupor; long-term application → transitory liver damage, reversible → liver enzyme blood values should be monitored

I: Unknown

Milk Thistle/St. Mary's Thistle
Cardui mariae fructus
Silybum marianum L. (GAERTN.)

AA: Dyspeptic complaints; preparations for toxic liver diseases, supportive therapy for chronic inflammatory liver disease, cirrhosis of the liver
Silymarin, the active principle of milk thistle in commercial preparations with standardized content is used as an antidote for amanita poisoning.

D: 3-4 g crushed herb (1-2 teaspoon)/150 mL, 10-15 min, also cold maceration, heat to boiling point,
1 cup 3-4 times/day,
daily dose: 12-15 g,
commercial preparations equivalent to 200-400 mg silymarin, calculated as silybin

A: Acute complaints > 1 week or recurring illness:
Please consult medical practitioner.

C: Commercial preparations containing standardized extracts are recommended.
Do not use tea preparations of the herb as an antidote for amanita poisoning.

CI: Unknown

AE: Unknown

I: Unknown

Mint Oil

Menthae arvensis aetheroleum
Mentha arvensis L. var. *piperascens* MALINV.

AA: **Internal:** Functional gastrointestinal complaints with tympanites, gallbladder disorders, catarrhs of the upper respiratory tract
External: Myalgia and neuralgic ailments

D: **Internal:** Average daily dose: 3-6 drops
Inhalation: 3-4 drops in hot water
External: Rub a few drops on the affected area;
mint oil in oily and semisolid preparations 5-10 percent essential oil, nose ointments 1-5 percent essential oil

A: Acute complaints > 1 week or recurring illness:
Please consult medical practitioner.

CI: **Internal:** Occlusion of the biliary ducts, gallbladder inflammation and severe liver damage, biliary colics due to the possible cholagogic effect for gallstone sufferers
External: Preparations containing the oil should not be applied directly to mucosa and wounds and not to the faces of infants or small children, particularly not in the nasal area; not for inhalation; → glottal spasm or bronchial spasm up to asthmalike attacks or even possible respiratory failure

AE: Gastric complaints

I: Unknown

Motherwort/Lion's Tail
Leonuri cardiacae herba
Leonurus cardiaca L.

AA: Nervous cardiac disorders, supportive therapy for hyper-thyroidism

D: 2-4.5 g (2-4 teaspoons)/150 mL, 10 min,
as a cure: 1 cup/day for 2-4 weeks, slightly tepid
daily dose: 4.5 g

A: Acute complaints > 1 week or recurring illness:
Please consult medical practitioner.

CI: Pregnancy

AE: Unknown; higher doses may lead to nausea, abdominal pains, blood in stool, excessive thirst.

I: Unknown

Mugwort/Common Wormwood
Artemisiae herba
Artemisia vulgaris L.

| ⚀ | 🚫 |

AA: Loss of appetite, gastrointestinal complaints; delayed or irregular menstruation; and worm infestations

D: Herb: 0.5-2 g (1-2 teaspoon)/150 mL, 10 min,
1 cup 2-3 times/day
pulverized herb: 1 knife tip (pinch) 5-6 times/day

C: Efficacy not proven; therapeutic use not recommended

CI: Pregnancy (abortive) and lactation

AE: Sensitization through skin contact

I: Unknown

Mullein Flower/Verbascum Flower
Verbasci flos
Verbascum densiflorum BERTOL, *V. phlomoides* L.

AA: Catarrh of respiratory tract

D: Approx. 1 g (1 teaspoon)/150 mL, 10-15 min,
1 cup 3-4 times/day,
daily dose 3-4 g

A: Acute complaints > 1 week or recurring illness:
Please consult medical practitioner.

C: Store protected from light and moisture; also used as orna-mental herb

CI: Unknown

AE: Unknown

I: Unknown

Myrrh/Myrrh Tincture
Myrrha, Myrrhae tinctura
Commiphora myrrha (NEES) ENGLER

AA: Mild inflammations of mouth, throat, and pharyngeal mucosa; sore gums due to wearing dentures; pediatrics: thrush

D: 2-3 times/day undiluted tincture, painted on;
cleansing and gargle: 5-10 drops of tincture in a glass of water *(Commission E)* or 30 to 60 drops in a glass of warm water; dental powders: 10 percent of powdered resin

A: Acute complaints > 1 week or recurring illness:
Please consult medical practitioner.

C: Undiluted application may cause transient mild burning and/ or sense of taste may be irritated

CI: Pregnancy

AE: Unknown

I: Unknown

Neem
Antelaeae azadirachtae cortex, folium
Azadirachta indica A. JUSS (syn. *Antelaea azadirachta* L.)

AA: Inflammatory and febrile diseases (including malaria and leprosy, although unconfirmed); dyspeptic complaints and worm infestation

D: Liquid tincture

A: Acute complaints > 1 week or recurring illness:
Please consult medical practitioner.

C: Efficacy not sufficiently proven

CI: Unknown

AE: Unknown with indicated usage

I: Unknown with indicated usage

Nettle Leaf and Herb
Urticae folium, U. herba
Urtica dioica L., *U. urens* L.

AA: **Internal:** Micturition problems in the case of prostate adenoma Stage I-II, cleansing therapy for inflammatory illness of derivative urinary tract, prophylaxis for gravel
External: Adjuvant treatment for rheumatic complaints

D: **Internal:** 4 g (4 teaspoons)/150 mL, 10 min,
also cold maceration;
as diuretic, 1 cup 2-3 times/day,
daily dose: 8-12 g
External: tincture, with ethanol 90 percent (1:10)

A: Acute complaints > 1 week or recurring illness:
Please consult medical practitioner.

C: Ensure sufficient fluid intake, minimum 2 L/day.

CI: Not useful for dehydration or edema due to reduced heart and renal activity

AE: Unknown

I: Unknown

Nettle Root
Urticae radix
Urtica dioica L., *U. urens* L.

AA: Micturition problems in the case of prostate adenoma Stage I-II

D: 1.5 g (1 teaspoon)/150 mL, boil for 1 min, 10 min,
1 cup 2-4 times/day,
daily dose: 4-6 g
dry extract: 120 mg 2 times/day

A: This herb only relieves the symptoms of an enlarged prostate without eliminating the enlargement itself. A specialist should be consulted at regular intervals.

C: Ensure sufficient fluid intake, minimum 2 L/day.

CI: Unknown

AE: Occasional, mild gastrointestinal complaints

I: Unknown

Oak Bark

Quercus cortex
Quercus robur L.

[⊛]

AA: **Internal:** Nonspecific acute diarrhea
External: Inflammatory skin diseases
Local: Mild inflammations of mouth, throat, and pharyngeal
mucosa; inflammations of the anal and genital area

D: **Internal:** 1 g (1/3 teaspoon)/150 mL,
cold maceration, boil for a few moments, 5-10 min, 1 cup 3
times/day,
daily dose: 3 g
External: Therapeutic bath: 500 g/100 L,
poultice: 20 g/1 L water, boil for 15-20 min
Local: Cleansing and gargle 20 g/1 L, boil for 15-20 min

A: For diarrhea > 3-4 days:
Please consult medical practitioner.
Not > 2-3 weeks

CI: No local application with extensive skin lesions;
therapeutic full baths with fever and infectious diseases, cardiac insufficiency Stage III-IV (NYHA), hypertonia Stage IV
(WHO): only after consulting medical practitioner

AE: Unknown

I: The absorption of alkaloids and other alkaline drugs may be
reduced or inhibited.

Oat Straw
Avenae stramentum
Avena sativa L.

AA: Inflammatory and seborrheic skin disorders, especially those accompanied by pruritus

D: Therapeutic bath: 50 g/100 L, 15-30 min

A: Acute complaints > 1 week or recurring illness:
Please consult medical practitioner.

C: Straw: Commission E: positive
Herb: Commission E: neutral

CI: No local application with extensive skin lesions; therapeutic full baths with fever and infectious diseases, cardiac insufficiency Stage III-IV (NYHA), hypertonia Stage IV (WHO): only after consulting medical practitioner.

AE: Unknown

I: Unknown

Olive Leaf

Oleae folium
Olea europaea L.

AA: In folk medicine for hypertonia, arteriosclerosis, rheumatism, and gout; diabetes mellitus; fever

D: 7-8 g (2 teaspoons)/150 mL, 30 min,
1 cup 3-4 times/day

A: Acute complaints > 1 week or recurring illness:
Please consult medical practitioner.

C: Efficacy has not been sufficiently documented; animal tests showed a hypotensive, antiarrhythmic, and spasmolytic effect on the smooth muscle of the intestine

CI: For safety reasons the therapeutic application of hypertonia cannot be recommended.

AE: Unknown

I: Unknown

Olive Oil
Olivae oleum
Olea europaea L.

AA: **Internal:** Traditionally used to lower LDL cholesterol level; application in discussion for cholangitis, inflammation of the gallbladder, flatulence, constipation, jaundice, gastrointestinal ulcers, and kidney stones
External: Wound care for mild burns, smoothing of crusts accompanying psoriasis and eczema, supportive treatment of rheumatism (massage oil), and sunburn
Local: Constipation (rectal)

D: **Internal:** 15-30 mL, 3 times/day with meals
External: Undiluted, in the production of liniments, ointments, soaps, poultices, and suspensions
Local: 100-500 mL at body temperature rectally

A: Acute complaints > 1 week or recurring illness:
Please consult medical practitioner.

C: Efficacy not proven; used as cooking oil

CI: Internal application not recommended to gallstone sufferers due to risk of colic

AE: Allergic skin reaction

I: Unknown

Onion
Alii cepae bulbus
Allium cepa L.

AA: **Internal:** Loss of appetite, arteriosclerosis prophylactic, vascular disease
External: insect bites, wounds, mild burns, boils, warts, and bruises

D: Therapeutic use of raw onion
Internal: onion tincture 4-5 teaspoons/day;
onion syrup 4-5 tablespoons/day,
daily dose: 50 g fresh onion or 20 g dried herb chopped or as pressed juice applied over a number of months
External: juice is spread or laid on as a poultice or in slices
onion pack: raw onions, cut into pieces or slices, put in cellulose bag, heated for 2 min, cooled down to 40°C, placed on aching ear

A: Acute complaints > 1 week or recurring illness:
Please consult medical practitioner.

CI: Unknown

AE: Intake of large quantities → stomach irritation and flatulence; frequent contact → rare allergic reactions (hand eczema)

I: Unknown

Parsley Herb and Root
Petroselini herba et radix
Petroselinum crispum (MILL.) NYM.

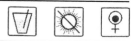

AA: Cleansing/irrigation therapy for nonspecific infections of the derivative urinary tract; prophylaxis and treatment of renal gravel

D: 2 g (1 teaspoon)/150 mL, 10-15 min,
1 cup 2-3 times/day,
daily dose: 6 g

A: Acute complaints > 1 week or recurring illness:
Please consult medical practitioner.

C: Higher doses of the essential parsley oil (e.g., as an abortifacient) or of preparations with high concentrations of the essential parsley oil → poisonings due to elevated contractility of the smooth muscle; for irrigation therapy ensure sufficient fluid intake, minimum 2 L/day

CI: Pregnancy; not useful for dehydration or edema due to reduced heart and renal activity

AE: Individual cases of skin and mucosa reactions; photosensitization possible, particularly for persons with light skin

I: Unknown

Passion Flower Herb/Maypop
Passiflorae herba
Passiflora incarnata L.

AA: Nervous agitation, mild insomnia, anxiety, nervous gastrointestinal complaints

D: 2 g (1 teaspoon)/150 mL, 10 min,
1 cup 2-4 times/day or 1-2 cups 30 min before going to sleep,
daily dose: 4-8 g

A: Acute complaints > 1 week or recurring illness:
Please consult medical practitioner.

C: Spasmolytic effect only with ethanolic extracts. The herb itself is rarely used for tea preparations; combinations with other sedative herbs maybe useful;
commercial preparations containing standardized extracts are also recommended.

CI: Unknown

AE: Unknown

I: Unknown

Peppermint Leaf
Menthae piperitae folium
Mentha × piperita L.

AA: Cramping pains in the gastrointestinal tract as well as gall-bladder and bilary duct

D: 1.5 g (2-3 teaspoons)/150 mL, 5-10 min,
1 cup 3-4 times/day
daily dose: 3-6 g

A: Acute > 1 week or regular recurring illness:
Please consult medical practitioner.

C: No risks with long-term treatment; flavoring agent

CI: For gallbladder or gallstones: only after consulting medical practioner → risk of colic

AE: Unknown

I: Unknown

Peppermint Oil
Menthae piperitae aetheroleum
Mentha × piperita L.

AA: **Internal:** Cramps of the upper gastrointestinal tract and biliary ducts, irritable colon; catarrhs of the respiratory tract
External: Myalgia and neuralgia; headache, common cold and cough
Local: Inflammation of mouth, throat, and pharyngeal mucosa

D: **Internal:** Average daily dose: 6-12 drops
Irritable colon: daily dose, 0.6 mL; single dose, 0.2 mL in enterically coated form
Inhalation: 3-4 drops in hot water
External: A few drops rubbed on the affected skin areas several (2-4) times/day, for young children: rub 5-15 drops on chest and back; semisolid and oily preparations: 5-20 percent, aqueous-ethanolic preparations: 5-10 percent, nose ointments: 1-5 percent

A: Acute complaints > 1 week or recurring illness:
Please consult medical practitioner.

C: Chronic gastric complaints → long-term therapy not recommended. Gallstones: Only with medical advice

CI: **Internal:** Occlusion of the biliary ducts, gallbladder inflammation and severe liver damage
External: Preparations containing the oil should not be applied to the faces of infants or small children, particularly not in the nasal area; not for inhalation; → glottal spasm or bronchial spasm up to asthmalike attacks or even possible respiratory failure

AE: Gastric complaints in susceptible persons

I: Unknown

Petasitis/Butterbur
Petasitidis rhizoma
Petasites hybridus (L.) GAERTN., MEY. & SCHERB.

AA: Supportive treatment of acute cramping pain of the gastrointestinal tract, in the derivative urinary tract, particularly in the presence of calculus; headache (migraine)

D: 1.2-2 g (2 teaspoons)/150 mL, 5-10 min,
1 cup 3 times/day
daily dose: Preparations equivalent to 4.5-7 g herb with a very low content of pyrrolizidine alkaloids (< 1 microgram)

A: Acute complaints > 1 week or recurring illness:
Please consult medical practitioner.

C: Not > 4-6 weeks/year; Therapeutic benefit controversial due to the presence of pyrrolizidine alkaloids with hepatotoxic and carcinogenic effect; herbal teas are not recommended; commercial preparations with a very low content of pyrrolizidine alkaloids are recommended; industrial manufacture of extracts virtually free of pyrrolizidine alkaloids is possible.

CI: Pregnancy and lactation

AE: High doses and long-term application → hepatotoxic, mutagenic, teratogenic, and carcinogenic effect

I: Unknown

Podophyllum/Mayapple/American Mandrake
Podophylli peltati rhizoma
Podophyllum peltatum L.

AA: **External:** Removal of genital warts; the resin is used only for removing pointed warts;
eczema

D: **Internal:** Obsolete as laxative
External: resin (podophyllin): warts, 5-25 percent solution or suspension; eczema, 0.1 percent ointment

A: Only with medical advice and supervision

C: The skin area to be treated should not exceed 25 square cm.

CI: Pregnancy, including external administration of the herb

AE: External administration of the herb over large skin areas may also lead to resorptive poisoning.

I: Unknown

Pokeweed/Phytolacca
Phytolaccae americanae radix
Phytolacca americana L.

AA: Immunomodulator

D: Single dose: 60-100 mg pulverized roots

A: Only with medical advice and supervision

C: Efficacy not proven; antiedemic and immune-stimulating effect has been demonstrated for the root; fruits used as a red coloring; herbal teas of both root and fruits unusual

CI: Pregnancy and lactation

AE: Overdose → severe intoxication, symptoms of poisoning include vomiting, diarrhea (sometimes bloody), severe thirst, dizziness, somnolence, hypotension, tachycardia, and in severe cases spasm and death through respiratory failure

I: Unknown

Pollen
Pollinae
diverse flowering plants

AA: Strengthening, invigoration in states of weakness, feebleness, debility, loss of appetite

D: Daily dose 30-40 g, commercial preparations equivalent; micronized pollen (< 10 μm) 3-4 g, commercial preparations equivalent

C: Herbal teas unusual

CI: Allergy to pollen

AE: Individual cases of gastrointestinal complaints

I: Unknown

Poplar Bud
Populi gemma
Populus tremula L.

AA: Superficial skin injuries, external hemorrhoids, frostbite, and sunburn

D: Semisolid preparations, equivalent to 20-30 percent of buds, daily dose: 5 g

A: Acute complaints > 1 week or recurring illness:
Please consult medical practitioner.

CI: Hypersensitivity to salicylates, propolis, and balm of Peru

AE: Occasional allergic skin reactions

I: Unknown

Poplar Leaf and Bark
Populi folium, P. cortex
Populus tremula L.

AA: Pain and rheumatism therapy; micturition complaints in the case of prostate adenoma Stages I-II

D: Dosage depends on the amount in combined preparations; dosage/efficacy ratio not proven;
daily dose: 10 g

A: This herb only relieves the symptoms of an enlarged prostate without eliminating the enlargement itself. A specialist should be consulted at regular intervals.

C: Poplar bark only available in combination with other herbs

CI: Hypersensitivity to salicylates

AE: Rare cases of hypersensitivity reactions

I: Unknown

Primula Flower and Root/
Cowslip Flower and Root
Primulae flos, P. radix
Primula veris L.

AA: Catarrh of respiratory tract; expectorant for cough and bronchitis

D: Flowers: Approx. 1 g (1 teaspoon)/150 mL, 10 min
1 cup several times/day,
daily dose: 2-4 g;
root: 0.5 g (¼ teaspoon)/150 mL, 10-15 min,
1 cup 1-3 times/day,
daily dose: 0.5-1.5 g

A: Acute complaints > 1 week or recurring illness:
Please consult medical practitioner.

C: Higher doses → renal irritations

CI: Allergy to cowslip, primroses

AE: Overdose → nausea, vomiting, gastric complaints, and diarrhea

I: Unknown

Pumpkin Seed
Cucurbitae semen
Cucurbita pepo L.

AA: Irritable bladder, micturition problems in the case of benign prostate adenoma Stages I-II

D: Herbal tea unusual; mornings and evenings 15-30 g (3-6 teaspoons) milled or ground with liquid;
commercial preparations containing standardized extracts equivalent to 15-30 g

A: Treatment should last several weeks up to months. This herb only relieves the symptoms of an enlarged prostate without eliminating the enlargement itself. A specialist should be consulted at regular intervals.

C: Ensure sufficient fluid intake, minimum 2 L/day.

CI: Unknown

AE: Unknown

I: Unknown

Puncture Vine-Burra Gokhru
Fructus tribuli
Tribulus terrestris L.

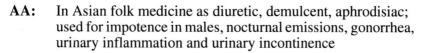

AA: In Asian folk medicine as diuretic, demulcent, aphrodisiac; used for impotence in males, nocturnal emissions, gonorrhea, urinary inflammation and urinary incontinence

D: Infusion 1 in 20: 3 times/day
Fluid extract: 10-30 drops

A: Acute complaints > 1 week or recurring illness:
Please consult medical practitioner.

C: Due to varying content of alkaloids (e.g., harmen, harman) the therapeutic use of this herb is not recommended.

Pygeum
Pygeum cortex
Pygeum africanum HOOK. F. (syn. *Prunus africana* (HOOK. f.)
KALKMAN)

AA: Symptomatic treatment of mild to moderate benign prostate hyperplasia

AE: Rarely cases of intestinal complaints, feeling of depletion, diarrhea, constipation, vertigo

D: Lipophilic extract: 100-200 mg

A: This herb only relieves the symptoms of an enlarged prostate without eliminating the enlargement itself. A specialist should be consulted at regular intervals.

C: Commercial preparations containing standardized extracts are recommended.

CI: Unknown

AE: Unknown

I: Unknown

Pyrethrum Flower/
Dalmatian Insect Flower
Pyrethri flos, Chrysanthemi cinerariifolii flos
Tanacetum cinerariifolium (TREVIR.) SCH. BIP.

AA: For head lice, crab lice, body lice, and their nits

D: **External:** liquid extract 0.3-0.5 percent, rinse after use
In commercial preparations (solution, spray, shampoo) according to package insert

C: Pyrethrins possess only limited toxicity for humans; doses up to 2 g of the flowers are nontoxic.
Contact with insecticide → paralysis of nervous system of arthropods; no acquired resistance for insects

CI: Unknown

AE: Minor sensitization tendency; signs of poisoning: headache, ringing in the ears, nausea, paresthesia, respiratory disturbances, and other neurotoxic symptoms

I: Unknown

Raspberry Leaf
Rubi idaei folium
Rubus idaeus L.

AA: Diseases and complaints of the gastrointestinal tract, the respiratory tract, the cardiovascular system, and the mouth and throat area

D: 1.5 g (2 teaspoons)/150 mL, 5 min,
1 cup 2-3 times/day

A: Acute complaints > 1 week or recurring illness:
Please consult medical practitioner.

C: Efficacy not proven, no risks, safe when used as ornamental and flavor-enhancing herb and in indicated doses; ingredient of diet drinks, in fruit tea mixtures

CI: Unknown

AE: Unknown

I: Unknown

Red Clover
Trifolii pratensis flos
Trifolium pratense L.

AA: **Internal:** For coughs and respiratory conditions; particularly whooping cough
External: Treatment of chronic skin conditions such as psoriasis and eczema

D: Infusion: 4 g up to 3 times/day
Liquid extract (1:1): 1.5-3 mL 3 times/day

A: Acute complaints > 1 week or recurring illness:
Please consult medical practitioner.

CI: Unknown

AE: Unknown

I: Unknown

Restharrow/Cammock
Ononidis radix
Ononis spinosa L.

AA: Irrigation therapy for inflammatory diseases of the lower urinary tract; prophylaxis and treatment of renal gravel

D: 2-2.5 g (1 scant teaspoon)/150 mL, 20-30 min,
1 cup 3-4 times/day,
daily dose: 6-12 g

A: Acute complaints > 1 week or recurring illness:
Please consult medical practitioner.

C: Ensure sufficient liquid intake, minimum 2 L/day

CI: Not useful for dehydration or edema due to reduced heart and renal activity

AE: Unknown

I: Unknown

Rhatany Root/Peruvian Rhatany
Ratanhiae radix
Krameria lappacea (DOMB.) BURD. et SIMP.
(syn. *K. triandra* RIUZ et PAV.)

AA: Mild inflammation of mouth, throat, and pharyngeal mucosa

D: 1.5 g (1/3 teaspoon)/150 mL, 10-15 min, 1 cup 3 times/day;
warm decoction for gargle and cleansing, 2-3 times/day;
tincture: 5-10 drops to a glass of warm water;
for painting on: 2-3 times/day undiluted tincture

A: Acute complaints > 1 week or recurring illness:
Please consult medical practitioner.

C: Ingredient in mouth spray, toothpaste

CI: Known allergy to preparations containing rhatany

AE: Internal administration → digestive complaints, rare cases of
allergic mucous membrane reactions

I: Unknown

Rhubarb Root
Rhei radix
Rheum palmatum L., *R. officinale* BAILL.

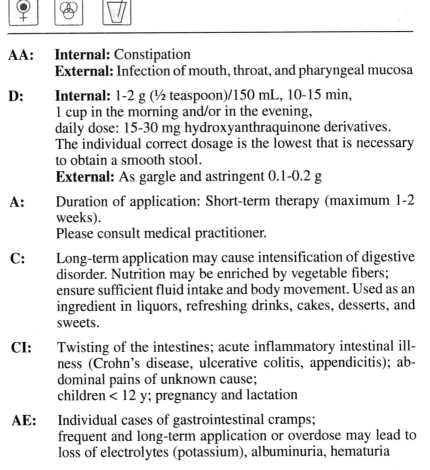

AA: **Internal:** Constipation
External: Infection of mouth, throat, and pharyngeal mucosa

D: **Internal:** 1-2 g (½ teaspoon)/150 mL, 10-15 min,
1 cup in the morning and/or in the evening,
daily dose: 15-30 mg hydroxyanthraquinone derivatives.
The individual correct dosage is the lowest that is necessary
to obtain a smooth stool.
External: As gargle and astringent 0.1-0.2 g

A: Duration of application: Short-term therapy (maximum 1-2
weeks).
Please consult medical practitioner.

C: Long-term application may cause intensification of digestive
disorder. Nutrition may be enriched by vegetable fibers;
ensure sufficient fluid intake and body movement. Used as an
ingredient in liquors, refreshing drinks, cakes, desserts, and
sweets.

CI: Twisting of the intestines; acute inflammatory intestinal illness (Crohn's disease, ulcerative colitis, appendicitis); abdominal pains of unknown cause;
children < 12 y; pregnancy and lactation

AE: Individual cases of gastrointestinal cramps;
frequent and long-term application or overdose may lead to
loss of electrolytes (potassium), albuminuria, hematuria

I: Deprivation of potassium → effect of cardioactive glycosides
↑, influence on the effect of antiarrhythmics

Roman Chamomile/ English Chamomile
Chamomillae romanae flos
Chamaemelum nobile (L.) ALL.

◎	⚲

AA: **Internal:** Feeling of repletion, flatulence, inflammation and spasms of the gastrointestinal tract
External: Eczema, wounds, skin inflammations
Local: Inflammation of mouth, throat, and pharyngeal mucosa

D: **Internal:** 2-3 g (2-3 teaspoons)/150 mL, 10 min, 1 cup 3-4 times/day
External: Ointment (3-10 percent herb), 1-2 times/day
Bath additive, 50 g/10 L water
Local: Decoction (3-10 percent herb), gargle and cleansing, several times/day

A: Acute complaints > 1 week or recurring illness:
Please consult medical practitioner.

C: Avoid eye area. Efficacy not proven. When used as ornamental herb, small potential for sensitization

CI: Pregnancy; hypersensitivity to Asteraceae; no local application with extensive skin lesions; therapeutic full baths with fever and infectious diseases, cardiac insufficiency Stage III-IV (NYHA), hypertonia Stage IV (WHO): only after consulting medical practitioner

AE: Unknown

I: Unknown

Rose Hips/Dog Rose
Rosae pseudofructus, Rosae pseudofructus cum fructibus
Rosa canina L., *R. pendulina* L.

⊙

AA: Prophylaxis and treatment of colds and flu, vitamin C deficiency (fresh fruits); minor complaints of gastrointestinal, biliary, and renal tracts

D: 2-5 g (1-2 teaspoons)/150 mL, 10-15 min, 1 cup several times/day

A: Acute complaints > 1 week or recurring illness: Please consult medical practitioner.

C: Efficacy not proven, no risks; vitamin C content is low and decreases quickly; ingredient of jams, compotes, juices, and desserts

CI: Unknown

AE: Unknown

I: Unknown

Rosemary Leaf
Rosmarini folium
Rosmarinus officinalis L.

⚥

AA: **Internal:** Dyspeptic complaints
External: Supportive therapy for rheumatic conditions, hypotonic circulatory disorders

D: **Internal:** 2 g (1 teaspoon)/150 mL, 15 min, 1 cup 3-4 times/day
External: Bath additive: 50 g/100 L water

A: Acute complaints > 1 week or recurring illness: Please consult medical practitioner.

C: Spice in food and in food industry

CI: Pregnancy

AE: Individual cases of contact allergies

I: Unknown

Saffron
Croci stigma
Crocus sativus L.

AA: In folk medicine as sedative for spasms and asthma; aromatic and flavor-enhancing herb

D: Maximum daily dose: 1.5 g (3 teaspoons)

A: Acute complaints > 1 week or recurring illness:
Please consult medical practitioner.

C: Efficacy not proven; risks with daily dose > 1.5 g
Spice; used as coloring agent in cakes, liqueurs, cosmetics, and pharmaceuticals industries

CI: Pregnancy

AE: Higher doses (> 5 g) → reactions, such as vomiting, uterine bleeding, diarrhea, yellowing of skin and mucosa
Lethal poisoning could occur with overdoses or through the abuse of larger doses as an abortifacient (abortive dosage approximately 10 g, lethal dosage approximately 12- 20 g).

I: Unknown

Sage/Red Sage
Salviae folium
Salvia officinalis L.

AA: **Internal:** Dyspeptic complaints, excessive perspiration
Local: Inflammation of mouth, throat, and pharyngeal mucosa, such as gingivitis and sore gums due to wearing dentures

D: **Internal:** 1.5 g (1 teaspoon)/150 mL, 10-15 min,
1 cup 2-4 times/day,
daily dose: 4-6 g herb, respectively 0.1-0.3 g essential oil
Local: Gargle and cleansing: 2.5 g/100 mL,
respectively 2-3 drops of essential oil/100 mL,
ethanolic tincture: 5 g/150 mL, several times/day;
paint on mucosa: undiluted ethanolic extract

A: Acute complaints > 1 week or recurring illness:
Please consult medical practitioner.

C: Long-term intake of ethanolic extracts of the herb or the essential oil → epileptiform convulsions

CI: Ethanolic extracts of the herb or the essential oil during pregnancy

AE: Unknown

I: Unknown

Sandalwood
Santali albi lignum
Santalum album L.

AA: Supportive therapy for infections of the derivative urinary tract

D: Daily dose: 10-20 g, respectively 1.0-1.5 g essential oil

A: Without medical advice and control, not > 6 weeks

C: Application of isolated sandalwood oil in a coating resistant to gastric juices

CI: Diseases of the renal parenchyma

AE: Skin itching, nausea, gastrointestinal complaints, and hematuria

I: Unknown

Sarsaparilla
Sarsaparillae radix
Smilax spp.

AA: In folk medicine for skin diseases, psoriasis, and resulting symptoms, rheumatic complaints, renal diseases, as a diuretic and diaphoretic

D: 1-5 g/150 mL, boil for 10 min,
1 cup with meals 3 times/day
Cold water extract: 2 teaspoons/ 250 mL cold water, 10-15 h, filter, drink warmed 500 mL mornings and evenings
Powder: daily dose: 0.3-1.5 g
Tincture: daily dose 5-15 g
Liquid extract (1:1, 20 percent ethanol, 10 percent glycerol): daily dose: 8-15 mL

A: Acute complaints > 1 week or recurring illness:
Please consult medical practitioner.

C: Efficacy not proven; no risks

CI: Unknown

AE: Diarrhea with vomiting, irritation of stomach and mucosa as well as renal irritation

I: Concomitant administration examples:
cardioactive glycosides or bismuth: absorption increased
hypnotics: elimination accelerated

Sassafras
Sassafras lignum
Sassafras albidum (NUTT.) NEES

AA: In folk medicine, used to be an ingredient of "blood-purify-ing tea" for skin disorders, catarrh, rheumatism, syphilis

A: Acute complaints > 1 week or recurring illness:
Please consult medical practitioner.

C: Efficacy not proven
Neither the herb nor its volatile oil should be administered or applied due to the carcinogenic effect of safrole.

CI: Pregnancy, lactation

AE: Unknown

I: Unknown

Saw Palmetto
Sabal fructus
Serenoa repens (BARTR.) SMALL

AA: Micturition problems, irritable bladder in the case of prostate adenoma Stage I-II

D: Daily dose: 1-2 g of herb or 20 mg lipophilic herb extract in 1-2 single doses

A: This herb only relieves the symptoms of an enlarged prostate without eliminating the enlargement itself. A specialist should be consulted at regular intervals.

C: Commercial preparations containing standardized extracts are recommended.

CI: Unknown

AE: Individual cases of gastrointestinal complaints

I: Unknown

Schisandra
Schisandrae fructus
Schisandra chinensis (TURCZ.) BAILL.

🚫

AA: In TCM for enuresis, nightly ejaculation, coughs, chronic diarrhea, dyspnea, insomnia, spontaneous outbreaks of sweating,
hepatitis, neurasthenia, intestinal inflammation, and anxiety

D: Powder/tincture/extract: daily dose: 1.5-6 g

A: Acute complaints > 1 week or recurring illness:
Please consult medical practitioner.

C: Efficacy not yet proven; variety of indications

CI: Unknown

AE: Unknown

I: Unknown

Seneca Root/Senega Root/ Snakeroot/Rattlesnake Root
Polygalae radix
Polygala senega L.

⊕

AA: Catarrh of respiratory tract, traditionally used as expectorant for bronchitis with minimum expectoration, tracheitis

D: 0.5 g (1 teaspoon equivalent to 3-4 g)/150 mL,
cold maceration, heat to boiling point, 10 min,
1 cup 2-3 times/day,
in serious cases every 2 h, under close observation for adverse effects
Daily dose: 1.5-3 g

A: Acute complaints > 1 week or recurring illness:
Please consult medical practitioner.

CI: Pregnancy

AE: Long-term application → gastrointestinal irritations; overdoses → nausea, diarrhea, gastric complaints, queasiness

I: Unknown

Senna
Sennae folium
Cassia senna L., *C. angustifolia* VAHL.

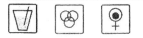

AA: Constipation

D: 0.5-2 g (½-1½ teaspoons)/150 mL, 10-15 min, 1 cup in the
          morning and/or in the evening,
          daily dose: 20-30 mg hydroxyanthraquinone derivatives
          The individual correct dosage is the lowest that is necessary
          to obtain a smooth stool.

A: Short-term therapy (maximum 1-2 weeks).
          Please consult medical practitioner.

C: Effect occurs after 10-12 hours. Long-term application may
          cause intensification of digestive disorders. Nutrition may be
          enriched by vegetable fibers; ensure sufficient fluid intake
          and body movement.

CI: Twisting of the intestines; acute inflammatory intestinal ill-
          ness (Crohn's disease, ulcerative colitis, appendicitis);
          abdominal pains of unknown cause;
          children < 12 y; pregnancy and lactation

AE: Individual cases of gastrointestinal cramps; frequent and
          long-term application or overdose may lead to loss of electro-
          lytes (potassium), albuminuria, hematuria

I: Deprivation of potassium → effect of cardioactive glycosides
          ↑, influences the effect of antiarrhythmics

Senna Pod
Sennae fructus acutifoliae (Alexandrine)
angustifoliae Sennae fructus (Tinnevelly)
Cassia senna L. (syn. *C. acutifolia* DEL.), *C. angustifolia* VAHL.

AA: Constipation

D: 1 g Alexandrine (1 teaspoon)
respectively 1-2 g Tinnevelly (1-2 teaspoons)/150 mL,
10 min, 1 cup in the morning and/or in the evening,
daily dose: 20-30 mg hydroxyanthraquinone derivatives
The individual correct dosage is the lowest that is necessary
to obtain a smooth stool.

A: Short-term therapy (maximum 1-2 weeks).
Please consult medical practitioner.

C: Effect occurs after 10 to 12 hours. Long-term application
may cause intensification of digestive disorders. Nutrition
should be enriched by vegetable fibers; ensure sufficient fluid
intake and body movement.

CI: First third of pregnancy: Only if vegetable fibers and dietary
changes have failed, with medical advice and supervision
Twisting of the intestines; acute inflammatory intestinal illness (Crohn's disease, ulcerative colitis, appendicitis);
abdominal pains of unknown cause;
children < 12 y; pregnancy (see above) and lactation

AE: Individual cases of gastrointestinal cramps;
frequent and long-term application or overdose
may lead to loss of electrolytes (potassium), albuminuria,
hematuria

I: Deprivation of potassium → effect of cardioactive glycosides
↑, influences the effect of antiarrhythmics

Shepherd's Purse/Caseweed Herb
Bursae pastoris herba
Capsella bursa-pastoris (L.) MEDIK.

⚲	�

AA: **Internal:** Mild menstrual irregularities such as menorrhagia and metrorrhagia
External: Nosebleeds, superficial, bleeding skin injuries

D: **Internal:** 3-5 g (2-3 teaspoons)/150 mL, 15 min,
1 cup 2-4 times/day between meals,
daily dose: 10-15 g
External: 3-5 g (2-3 teaspoons)/150 mL

A: For continuous bleeding please consult medical practitioner.

CI: Pregnancy

AE: Unknown

I: Unknown

Silverweed/Goose Gras
Anserinae herba
Potentilla anserina L.

AA: **Internal:** Adjuvant treatment of nonspecific, acute diarrhea; dysmenorrhea symptoms
Local: Topical treatment of inflammation of mouth, throat, and pharyngeal mucosa

D: **Internal:** 2 g (2 teaspoons)/150 mL, 10 min, 1 cup several times/day between meals, daily dose: 4-6 g
Local: Cleansing and gargle; *see* INTERNAL

A: For diarrhea > 3-4 days, please consult medical practitioner.

CI: Unknown

AE: Complaints connected with irritable stomach may increase.

I: Unknown

Slippery Elm Bark
Ulmi fulvae cortex
Ulmus rubra MÜHLENB.

☒·

AA: **Internal:** Soothes inflammations of mouth, throat, pharyn-geal, and gastrointestinal mucosa
External: Wounds, burns, skin diseases

D: **Internal:** Decoction: 4-16 mL/day
External: Coarsely ground herb used as poultice

A: Acute complaints > 1 week or recurring illness:
Please consult medical practitioner.

CI: Unknown

AE: Unknown

I: Unknown

Small-Flowered Willow Herb
Epilobii herba
Epilobium parviflorum SCHREB.

AA: Traditionally used with micturation problems in the case of prostate adenoma Stage I-II

D: 1.5-2 g (1-2 teaspoons)/150 mL, 10-15 min,
1 cup 2 times/day

A: Acute complaints > 1 week or recurring illness:
Please consult medical practitioner.

CI: Unknown

AE: Unknown

I: Unknown

Soybean Lecithin
Lecithinum ex soja
Glycine max (L.) MERR.

AA: Mild forms of hypercholesterolemia when dietary measures alone have failed

D: Daily dose: Total phospholipids in natural mixture equivalent to 3.5 g (phosphatidylcholine)

A: Acute complaints > 1 week or recurring illness: Please consult medical practitioner.

CI: Unknown

AE: Unknown

I: Unknown

Spanish Psyllium Seed/French Psyllium Seed
Psylli semen
Plantago afra L.

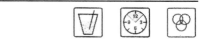

AA: Habitual or chronic constipation; supportive therapy for diarrhea and irritable bowel

D: 5-10 g dry seed (1-2 teaspoons)/150 mL, allow to soak, 200 mL liquid intake afterward;
daily dose: 10-30 g

A: With diarrhea > 3-4 days:
Please consult medical practitioner.

C: 30-60 min interval from intake of meals and other medication; ensure sufficient fluid intake, minimum 2 L/day.

CI: Pathological narrowing of gastrointestinal tract, risk of intestinal blockage; diabetes mellitus difficult to regulate

AE: Rare allergic reactions, especially with pulverized herb and liquid preparation

I: Simultaneous medication → absorption ↓; insulin-dependent diabetes → dose of insulin ↓

Spearmint Leaf
Menthae crispae folium
Mentha spicata L. ssp. *spicata*

☒

AA: **Local:** Oral antiseptic, in mouthwash, tooth care products, chewing gum (spearmint)
Internal: Stomachic, carminative, digestive aid, flatulence

D: **Internal:** 1-1.5 g (1 scant teaspoon)/150 mL, 10 min, 1 cup several times/day

A: For persistent complaints please consult medical practitioner.

CI: Unknown

AE: Unknown

I: Unknown

Speedwell
Veronicae herba
Veronica officinalis L.

AA: **Internal:** Complaints and symptoms of the respiratory tract
External: Inflammations of mouth, throat, and pharyngeal mucosa, promotion of wound healing, for chronic skin complaints, itching, and sweating of the feet

D: **Internal:** 1.5 (1 teaspoon)/150 mL, 10 min, 1 cup 2-3 times/day
External: Gargle, for lavage and poultice for ulcers 10-20 g/1 L water, boil for 10 min

A: Acute complaints > 1 week or recurring illness: Please consult medical practitioner.

C: Efficacy not sufficiently proven

CI: Unknown

AE: Unknown

I: Unknown

St. John's Wort
Hyperici herba
Hypericum perforatum L.

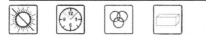

AA: **Internal:** Transient mild to moderate depression; psycho-vegetative disorders, anxiety, nervous restlessness; oil preparation for indigestion
External: Oil preparation for initial and follow-up treatment of sharp and blunt injuries and first-degree burns, myalgia

D: **Internal:** 2-4 g (2 teaspoons)/150 mL, 5-10 min, 1-2 cups regularly in the morning and in the evening; however, herbal teas are no longer recommended due to variation of natural product contents and the limited extractability of an aqueous decoction. Commercial preparations containing standardized extracts are recommended.
External: Application of the fatty oil, also in products containing other fatty oils at different concentrations

A: For more intensive symptoms:
Please consult medical practitioner.

C: Mood improvement may last up to 6 weeks; Due to strong influence of herb quality on extract quality, only herbs under controlled cultivation (GAP: good agricultural practices) should be used for extract preparation.

CI: Intensive UV radiation; do not use with prescription medications unless advised to do so by a physician, because of possible interactions.

AE: Possible photosensitization; pale-skinned persons should be cautious in using high doses.

I: Hypericum-containing preparations should not be administered together with

- digoxin,
- coumarinergic oral anticoagulants (e.g., phenprocoumon),

- cyclosporine,
- indinavir, and
- similar protease inhibitors.

Isolated cases of interaction have been reported with

- theophylline,
- oral contraceptives, and
- tricyclic antidepressants (amitryptiline).

Tea Tree Oil
Melaleucae aetheroleum
Melaleuca alternifolia CHEEL.

AA: **Internal:** In folk medicine for tonsillitis, pharyngitis, colitis, sinusitis
External: In folk medicine for mycosis of the nails, skin infections, ulcers, burns, acne, and insect bites
Local: In folk medicine for ulcers of the oral mucous membrane, gingivitis

D: **Internal/Local:** Currently, no reasonable dosages documented
External: Mycosis of the nail: undiluted;
acne: 5 percent in aqueous gel preparations

A: Acute complaints > 1 week or recurring illness:
Please consult medical practitioner.

C: Efficacy has not been proven; mainly used as ingredient in so-called natural cosmetics for skin care

CI: Unknown

AE: Allergic skin reactions; overdose (10 mL for a child) → several cases of poor coordination weakness and confusion, very high dose (approx. 70 mL) → coma

I: Unknown

Temoe Lawak/Javanese Turmeric
Curcumae xanthorrhizae rhizoma
Curcuma xanthorrhiza ROXB.

AA: Dyspeptic complaints, loss of appetite, stomachic and carminative

D: 0.5-1.0 g (1/3 teaspoon)/150 mL, 5-10 min,
1 cup 2-3 times/day between meals,
daily dose: 2 g

A: Acute complaints > 1 week or recurring illness:
Please consult medical practitioner.

CI: Do not use with obstructed biliary duct because of stimulating effect upon the biliary tract.
Gallstones: Only with medical advice → risk of colic

AE: Long-term therapy, overdose → gastric mucosa irritation possible

I: Unknown

Thuja/Arborvitae
Thujae occidentalis herba
Thuja occidentalis L.

| ⚲ | ✉ |

AA: **Internal:** Diuretic; fever and common cold, susceptibility to infections
External: Topical treatment of warts caused by viral infections

D: **Internal:** Tea preparations not recommended due to dosage difficulties because of the toxicity of the herb (thujone). Commercial preparations containing standardized extracts (with practically no thujone) should be used according to the package insert.
Extract (50 percent ethanol 1:1): 2 mL 3 times/day
External: Tincture (undiluted): maximum 0.5 g for application on skin

A: Acute complaints > 1 week or recurring illness:
Please consult medical practitioner.

C: Thuja extracts in compound preparations; overdose, particularly after misuse of the herb as an abortifacient → queasiness, vomiting, painful diarrhea, and mucous membrane hemorrhaging

CI: Pregnancy

AE: Unknown, if commercial preparations are used

I: Unknown, if commercial preparations are used

Thyme
Thymi herba
Thymus vulgaris L., *T. zygis* L.

AA: **Internal/External:** Symptoms of bronchitis, whooping cough, catarrh of upper respiratory tract
Local: Inflammation of mouth, throat, and pharyngeal mucosa

D: **Internal:** 1-2 g (1-2 teaspoons)/150 mL, 10-15 min,
1 cup several times/day,
daily dose: 10 g, containing 0.03 percent phenols
External: Poultice: 5 percent infusion,
full bath: 500 g/100 L
Local: Gargle and cleansing; for dosage *see* INTERNAL

A: Acute complaints > 1 week or recurring illness:
Please consult medical practitioner.

C: Combination with other expectorant herbs recommended

CI: No local application with extensive skin lesions; therapeutic full baths with fever and infectious diseases, cardiac insufficiency Stage III-IV (NYHA), hypertonia Stage IV (WHO): only after consulting medical practitioner.

AE: Unknown

I: Unknown

Tormentil
Tormentillae rhizoma
Potentilla erecta (L.) RÄUSCH.

AA: **Internal:** Nonspecific acute diarrhea
Local: Inflammation of mouth, throat, and pharyngeal mucosa, sore gums due to wearing dentures

D: **Internal:** 2-3 g (½ teaspoon)/150 mL,
cold maceration, heat to boiling point, 10-15 min,
1 cup 3 times/day,
average daily dose: 4-6 g
Local: Gargle and cleansing; for dosage *see* INTERNAL

A: For diarrhea > 3-4 days: Please consult medical practitioner.

CI: Do not use for diarrhea in babies and infants; consult medical practitioner immediately.

AE: Gastric complaints and vomiting in susceptible persons

I: Unknown

Turmeric
Curcumae longae rhizoma
Curcuma domestica VAL (syn. *C. longa* L.)

AA: Dyspeptic complaints, particularly feelings of fullness after meals and regular tympanites

D: 1.3 g (1 very scant teaspoon)/150 mL, 10-15 min, 1 cup 2 times/day between meals,
powder: 2-3 times/day after meals,
daily dose: 1.5-3 g
tincture (1:10): 10-15 drops 2-3 times/day

A: Acute complaints > 1 week or recurring illness:
Please consult medical practitioner.

C: Herbal teas unusual; commercial preparations containing standardized extracts are recommended.
Spice, particularly in curry powder

CI: Do not use with obstructed biliary duct because of stimulating effect upon the biliary tract.
Gallstones: Only with medical advice → risk of colic

AE: Long-term therapy, overdose → gastric mucosa irritation possible

I: Unknown

Uzara Root

Uzarae radix

Xysmalobium undulatum (L.) R. BR.

AA: Nonspecific acute diarrhea

D: Initial single dose:
Adults: 75 mg total glycosides (calculated as uzarin)
children: 15-30 mg total glycosides
infants: 1-2 times/day, 15 mg total glycosides
daily dose:
adults/children: 45-90 mg of total glycosides

A: For diarrhea > 3-4 days:
Please consult medical practitioner.

C: Herbal teas unusual; commercial preparations containing standardized extracts (tablets, drops, dose according to package inserts) are recommended.

CI: Therapy with cardioactive glycosides; do not use for diarrhea in babies and infants; immediately consult medical practitioner.

AE: Unknown

I: Unknown

Valerian Root, Tincture
Valerianae radix, V. tinctura
Valeriana officinalis L.

AA: **Internal:** Nervous restlessness and initial insomnia (problems in falling asleep); muscle relaxant
External: Muscle relaxation, mild sedative in therapeutic baths

D: **Internal:** Infusion 2-3 g (1 teaspoon)/150 mL, 10-15 min,
1 cup several times/day and before going to bed,
daily dose: 15 g
tincture: Several times/day 30-50 drops in water
plant juice: adults, 3 × 1 tablespoon; children, 3 × 1 teaspoon
External: Therapeutic full bath: 50 g/100 L,
volatile oil: 0.2 g/100 L

A: Periodically recurring illnesses, complaints, conditions:
Please consult medical practitioner.

C: Commercial preparations containing standardized extracts are recommended.

CI: No local application with extensive skin lesions; therapeutic baths with fever and infectious diseases, cardiac insufficiency Stage III-IV (NYHA), hypertonia Stage IV (WHO): only after consulting medical practitioner.

AE: Gastrointestinal complaints uncommon; contact allergies very uncommon

I: Unknown

Vervain
Verbenae herba
Verbena officinalis L.

⚲	◯

AA: **Internal:** Secretolytic with complaints of the upper respiratory tract; renal and derivative urinary tract complaints; to promote lactation; for rheumatic diseases
Local: Gargle for cold symptoms and for diseases of the oral and pharyngeal cavity

D: **Internal:** 1.5 g (1 teaspoon)/150 mL, 5-10 min, 1 cup up to 3 times/day
Local: Infusion: 5-20 g/1 L, 5-10 min

A: Acute complaints > 1 week or recurring illness: Please consult medical practitioner.

C: Efficacy not yet proven; secretolytic effect for catarrhs of the upper respiratory tract in compound preparations possible

CI: Pregnancy

AE: Unknown

I: Unknown

Walnut Leaf
Juglandis folium
Juglans regia L.

AA: Mild, superficial skin inflammations; excessive perspiration, for example, of hands and feet

D: 2-3 g (2-3 teaspoons)/150 mL, cold maceration, heat to boiling point for 15 min, for poultice and as bath additive

A: Acute complaints > 1 week or recurring illness: Please consult medical practitioner.

C: In compound preparations

CI: Unknown

AE: Unknown

I: Unknown

White Dead Nettle/Archangel
Lamii albi flos
Lamium album L.

AA: **Internal:** Catarrh of the upper respiratory tract, esp. as a mucolytic
External: Mild, superficial skin inflammations
Local: Mild inflammations of the oral and pharyngeal cavity; nonspecific leukorrhea

D: **Internal:** 1 g (2 teaspoons)/150 mL, 5 min,
1 cup 3 times/day,
daily dose: 3 g
External: Hip bath: 5 g
Local: Cleansing and gargle; for dosage *see* INTERNAL

A: Acute complaints > 1 week or recurring illness:
Please consult medical practitioner.

C: The traditional use of white deadnettle for leukorrhea needs to be reviewed.

CI: Unknown

AE: Unknown

I: Unknown

Wild Thyme/Mother of Thyme/Serpyllum
Serpylli herba
Thymus serpyllum L.

AA: **Internal:** Catarrh of the upper respiratory tract; feeling of fullness, flatulence
External: Acute and chronic conditions of the respiratory tract (full baths)

D: **Internal:** 1.5-2 g (1-2 teaspoons)/150 mL, 10 min,
as expectorant 1 cup several times/day,
as stomachic 1 cup before or after meals
External: Bath: 100 g/100 L water (equivalent to 4 g wild thyme oil)

A: Acute complaints > 1 week or recurring illness:
Please consult medical practitioner.

CI: Unknown; no local application with extensive skin lesions; therapeutic baths with fever and infectious diseases, cardiac insufficiency Stage III-IV (NYHA), hypertonia Stage IV (WHO): only after consulting medical practitioner

AE: Unknown

I: Unknown

Willow Bark

Salicis cortex
Salix purpurea L., *S. daphnoides* VIL. (among others)

AA: Febrile conditions, headaches, rheumatic conditions

D: 2-3 g (1 teaspoon)/150 mL, cold maceration,
heat to boiling point for 5 min,
1 cup 3-5 times/day,
daily dose: 6-12 g,
equivalent to 60-120 mg total salicin

A: Acute complaints > 1 week or recurring illness:
Please consult medical practitioner.

C: Also commercial preparations containing standardized extracts

CI: Hypersensitivity to salicylates

AE: Gastric complaints (tannin content); with hypersensitivity, allergic reactions possible

I: Unknown

Witch Hazel Bark/Hamamelis Bark
Hamamelidis cortex
Hamamelis virginiana L.

AA: **External/Local:** Minor skin injuries, local skin and mucosa inflammations, varicose veins, and hemorrhoids

D: **External/Local:**
Cleansing and poultice:
5-10 g (2-4 teaspoons)/250 mL
Gargle: 2-3 g (1-1½ teaspoons)/150 mL
Semisolid and liquid preparations: 5-10 percent herb

A: Acute complaints > 1 week or recurring illness:
Please consult medical practitioner.

C: Forms of commercial preparations: ointment, cream, gel, suppositories, and compound preparations using water and/or alcoholic extracts

CI: No local application with extensive skin lesions; therapeutic baths with fever and infectious diseases, cardiac insufficiency Stage III-IV (NYHA), hypertonia Stage IV (WHO): only after consulting medical practitioner.

AE: Unknown for external/local application

I: Unknown for external/local application

Witch Hazel Leaf/Hamamelis Leaf

Hamamelidis folium
Hamamelis virginiana L.

AA: **External/Local:** Minor skin injuries, local skin and mucosa inflammations, varicose veins, and hemorrhoids

D: **External/Local:**
Cleansing and poultice:
5-10 g (10-20 teaspoons)/250 mL
gargle: 2-3 g (4-6 teaspoons)/150 mL
semisolid and liquid preparations: 5-10 percent herb

A: Acute complaints > 1 week or recurring illness:
Please consult medical practitioner.

C: Forms of commercial preparations: ointment, cream, gel, suppositories, and compound preparations using water and/or alcoholic extracts

CI: No local application with extensive skin lesions; therapeutic baths with fever and infectious diseases, cardiac insufficiency Stage III-IV (NYHA), hypertonia Stage IV (WHO): only after consulting medical practitioner

AE: Unknown

I: Unknown

Wormwood/Absinthe
Absinthii herba
Artemisia absinthium L.

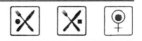

AA: Loss of appetite, dyspeptic complaints, cramplike functional disturbances of biliary ducts

D: 1.5 g (1 teaspoon)/150 mL, 10 min,
1 cup 2 times/day,
appetite enhancer → 30 min before meals
dyspeptic complaints → after meals,
daily dose: 2-3 g

A: Acute complaints > 1 week or recurring illness:
Please consult medical practitioner; no long-term application

C: Use of volatile oils and spirituous herb extracts for the manufacture of alcoholic drinks is forbidden in many countries because of possible health problems.
Combination with other bitters or aromatics may be advantageous.

CI: Pregnancy

AE: Unknown, with the proper administration of designated therapeutic dosages. Long-term application and/or overdose → vomiting, stomach and intestinal cramp, headache, dizziness, and disturbances of the central nervous system due to the herb's possible thujone content

I: Unknown with indicated usage

Yarrow/Milfoil
Millefolii herba
Achillea millefolium L.

✕

AA: **Internal:** Loss of appetite as aromatic bitter,
increase of biliary secretion, dyspeptic complaints such as
mild disturbances of the gastrointestinal tract (inflammation,
diarrhea, flatulence, cramps)
External: Hip bath for female functional lower abdominal
complaints;
palliative for liver disorders;
healing agent for inflammatory skin diseases

D: **Internal:** 2-4 g (1-2 teaspoons)/150 mL, 10 min,
1 cup 3-4 times/day between meals
External: 100 g/100 L, 20 min

A: Acute complaints > 1 week or recurring illness:
Please consult medical practitioner.

CI: Hypersensitivity to yarrow and other Asteraceae; no local application with extensive skin lesions; therapeutic baths with
fever and infectious diseases, cardiac insufficiency Stage III-
IV (NYHA), hypertonia Stage IV (WHO): only after consulting medical practitioner

AE: Rare cases of hypersensitivity reactions

I: Unknown

Yellow Bedstraw Herb/Lady's Bedstraw
Galii veri herba
Galium verum L.

○

AA: **Internal:** Uriniparous, uriniferous, to increase urinary excretion

External: Poorly healing wounds, to promote wound healing

D: **Internal/External:** 4-5 g (2 teaspoons)/150 mL,
10 min, also cold maceration,
1 cup 2-3 times/day,
also for moist poultice

C: Efficacy not proven; the herb may be considered obsolete.

CI: No local application with extensive skin lesions; therapeutic baths with fever and infectious diseases, cardiac insufficiency Stage III-IV (NYHA), hypertonia Stage IV (WHO): only after consulting medical practitioner

AE: Unknown

I: Unknown

Yellow Chaste Weed/Everlasting Flower
Helichrysi flos
Helichrysum arenarium (L.) MOENCH

AA: Dyspeptic complaints; as an adjunct in the treatment of chronic cholecystitis and convulsive gallbladder diseases

D: Approx. 1 g (1 teaspoon)/150 mL, 5-10 min, 1 cup 3-4 times/day, average daily dose: 3 g

A: Acute complaints > 1 week or recurring illness: Please consult medical practitioner.

C: Also used as ornamental herb

CI: Do not use with obstructed biliary duct because of stimulating effect upon the biliary tract.
Gallstones: Only with medical advice → risk of colic
Hypersensitivity to Asteraceae

AE: Unknown

I: Unknown

Yohimbe
Yohimbehe cortex
Pausinystalia yohimbe (K. SCHUM.) PIERRE ex BEILLE

🚫

AA: Sexual disorders, as an aphrodisiac, as well as for debility and exhaustion

D: According to package insert in commercial preparations

A: Acute complaints > 1 week or recurring illness:
Please consult medical practitioner.

C: Forms of commercial preparations: Tablets and various compound preparations

CI: Liver and renal diseases

AE: Agitation, sleeplessness, anxiety, tremor, tachycardia, elevated blood pressure, queasiness, vomiting, exanthema;
overdose → salivation, mydriasis, evacuation, loss of blood pressure, disorders of the cardiac impulse-conducting system with negative ionotropic effect. Death can occur through cardiac failure.

I: Interactions with psychopharmacological herbs have been reported.

Zedoary
Zedoariae rhizoma
Curcuma zedoaria (CHRISTM.) ROSC.

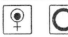

AA: Colics, cramps, gastric conditions, and digestive complaints

D: 1-1.5 (1/3 teaspoon)/150 mL, 3-5 min,
also cold maceration,
1 cup 3 times/day

A: Acute complaints > 1 week or recurring illness:
Please consult medical practitioner

C: Efficacy not yet proven; no risks; component of Swedish bitters

CI: Pregnancy

AE: Unknown

I: Unknown

List of Medicinal Herbs

ENGLISH-LATIN

Agrimony — *Agrimonia eupatoria* L.

Angelica root, European angelica root — *Angelica archangelica* L.

Anise, aniseed — *Pimpinella anisum* L.

Arnica flower, leopard's bane — *Arnica montana* L.

Artichoke leaf — *Cynara scolymus* L.

Ashwagandha — *Withania somnifera* DUNAL

Astragalus — *Astragalus membranaceus* (FISCH.) BGE. var. *mongolicus* (BGE.) HSIAO

Avocado oil — *Persea americana* MILL.

Balm leaf, lemon balm, melissa — *Melissa officinalis* L.

Barbados aloe, Curaçao aloe — *Aloe barbadensis* MILL.

Bearberry leaf — *Arctostaphylos uva-ursi* (L.) SPRENGEL

Bilberry, blueberry — *Vaccinium myrtillus* L.

Bilberry leaf, blueberry leaf — *Vaccinium myrtillus* L.

Birch leaf — *Betula pubescens* EHRH., *B. pendula* ROTH.

Bitter orange peel — *Citrus aurantium* L. ssp. *aurantium*

Black cohosh — *Cimicifuga racemosa* (L.) NUTT.

Black knotweed, hogweed — *Polygonum aviculare* L.

Black or European elder flower — *Sambucus nigra* L.

Blackberry leaf — *Rubus fruticosus* L.

Blackthorn flower — *Prunus spinosa* L.

Blackthorn fruit — *Prunus spinosa* L.

Blessed thistle, holy thistle — *Cnicus benedictus* L.

Blond psyllium husk/seed, Indian plantago, ispaghula — *Plantago ovata* FORSK.

Boldo leaf — *Peumus boldus* MOL.

Buckbean, bogbean — *Menyanthes trifoliata* L.

Buckthorn — *Rhamnus cathartica* L.

Buckwheat herb	*Fagopyrum esculentum* MOENCH
Bugleweed, gypsywort	*Lycopus europaeus* L., *L. virginicus* L.
Burdock, great burdock	*Arctium lappa* L.
Butcher's-broom, box holly	*Ruscus aculeatus* L.
Calamus, sweet flag	*Acorus calamus* L.
Calendula, marigold flower	*Calendula officinalis* L.
Cape aloe	*Aloe ferox* MILL.
Caraway	*Carum carvi* L.
Cardamom	*Elettaria cardamomum* (L.) MATON
Carline thistle	*Carlina acaulis* L.
Cascara sagrada, sacred bark, chittem bark	*Frangula purshiana* (DC.) COOP.
Cat's claw, uña de gato	*Uncaria tomentosa* (WILLD.) DC.
Cayenne pepper, chilies, tabasco pepper	*Capsicum frutescens* L.
Chamomile, German chamomile flower	*Matricaria recutita* L.
Chaste tree	*Vitex agnus-castus* L.
Chicory, succory	*Cichorium intybus* L.
Chinese cassia/cassia	*Cinnamomum aromaticum* NEES.
Chinese or Korean ginseng root	*Panax ginseng* C. A. MEY.
Cinnamon bark, Ceylon cinnamon	*Cinnamomum ceylanicum* BLUME, *C. verum* J. S. PRESL.
Cloves, clove oil	*Syzygium aromaticum* (L.) MERR. et L. M. PERRY
Coltsfoot leaf, tussilago leaf	*Tussilago farfara* L.
Comfrey leaf, herb	*Symphytum officinale* L.
Comfrey root	*Symphytum officinale* L.
Common centaury, centaury herb	*Centaurium erythraea* RAFN.
Coriander	*Coriandrum sativum* L.
Corn silk	*Zea mays* L.
Couch grass, quack grass	*Agropyron repens* (L.) P. BEAUV.
Cundurango, eagle vine	*Marsdenia cundurango* Reich. f.
Damiana	*Turnera diffusa* WILLD. ex SCHULT. ssp. *gigantea*, *Turnera diffusa* var. *aphrodisiaca* (KINGDON-WARD) URBAN
Dandelion root and herb	*Taraxacum officinale* WEB.
Devil's claw	*Harpagophytum procumbens* (BURCH.) DC.
Dill	*Anethum graveolens* L. ssp. *graveolens*
Dong quai, danggui	*Angelica sinensis* (OLIV.) DIELS
Drosera, sundew herb	*Drosera madagascariensis* DC., *D. peltata* SMITH
Early goldenrod	*Solidago gigantea* AIT. ssp. *gigantea*

Echinacea pallida root	*Echinacea pallida* (NUTT.) NUTT.
Echinacea purpurea herb	*Echinacea purpurea* (L.) MOENCH
Eleuthero, Siberian ginseng	*Eleutherococcus senticosus* MAXIM.
English plantain, ribwort	*Plantago lanceolata* L.
Ephedra herb, ma huang	*Ephedra sinica* STAPF, *E. shennungiana* TANG
Eucalyptus	*Eucalyptus globulus* LABILL.
Eucalyptus oil	*Eucalyptus globulus* LABILL.
European goldenrod	*Solidago virgaurea* L.
European mistletoe	*Viscum album* L.
Eyebright herb	*Euprasia stricta* WOLFF ex. J. F. LEHM.
Fennel	*Foeniculum vulgare* MILL., var. *vulgare,* var. *dulce*
Fenugreek seed	*Trigonella foenum-graecum* L.
Feverfew herb	*Tanacetum parthenium* (L.) SCHULTZ. BIP.
Frangula bark, buckthorn bark	*Rhamnus frangula* L.
Fucus, kelp	*Fucus vesiculosus* L.
Fumitory herb, earth smoke	*Fumaria officinalis* L.
Galangal, Chinese ginger, galanga	*Alpinia officinarum* HANCE
Garlic, garlic oil	*Allium sativum* L.
Gentian	*Gentiana lutea* L.
Ginger, ginger root	*Zingiber officinale* ROSC.
Ginkgo, ginkgo biloba extract	*Ginkgo biloba* L.
Goldenseal, hydrastis	*Hydrastis canadensis* L.
Grape seed	*Vitis vinifera* L.
Great burnet saxifrage, saxifrage	*Pimpinella major* (L.) HUDS., *P. saxifraga* L.
Greater celandine	*Chelidonium majus* L.
Greek sage leaf	*Salvia triloba* L. FIL.
Guggul, guggal	*Commiphora mukul* (HOOK. ex STOCKS) ENGL.
Haronga, harungana bark, leaf	*Harungana madagascariensis* LAM. ex POIR.
Hawthorn herb with flower; haw, white thorn	*Crataegus monogyna* JAQC.
Hayseed flower	Graminaceae, meadow flowers
Heartsease, wild pansy	*Viola tricolor* L.
Hemp nettle	*Galeopsis segetum* NECKER
Henna	*Lawsonia inermis* L.
Herniary, rupturewort	*Herniaria glabra* L.
Hibiscus flower, Jamaica sorrel, roselle	*Hibiscus sabdariffa* L.
Hops	*Humulus lupulus* L.
Horehound, hoarhound	*Marrubium vulgare* L.

Horny goat weed, barrenwort	*Epimedium* spp.
Horse chestnut seed	*Aesculus hippocastanum* L.
Horsetail	*Equisetum arvense* L.
Iceland moss	*Cetraria islandica* (L.) ACH.
Indian frankincense	*Boswellia carteri* BIRDW.
Indian olibanum tree	*Boswellia serrata* ROXB. ex COLEBR.
Ipecacuanha root, ipecac	*Psychotria ipecacuanha* (BROT.) STOKES
Ivy, English ivy	*Hedera helix* L.
Java citronella oil	*Cymbopogon winterianus* IOWITT.
Java tea	*Orthosiphon aristatus* (BLUME) MIQ.
Juniper berry	*Juniperus communis* L.
Khella, visnaga	*Ammi visnaga* (L.) LAM.
Lady's mantle, lion's foot	*Alchemilla xanthochlora* ROTHM.
Lavender flower	*Lavandula angustifolia* MILL.
Lavender oil	*Lavandula angustifolia* MILL.
Licorice root, glycyrrhiza	*Glycyrrhiza glabra* L.
Linden flower, lime tree flower	*Tilia cordata* MILL., *T. platyphyllos* SCOP., *T. vulgaris* HEYNE
Linseed, flaxseed	*Linum usitatissimum* L.
Lovage root	*Levisticum officinale* KOCH
Lycopodium herb, club moss	*Lycopodium clavatum* L.
Mallow leaf and flower	*Malva neglecta* WALLR., *Malva sylvestris* ssp. *mauritiana* (L.) BOISS. ex COUT
Manna	*Fraxinus ornus* L.
Marshmallow leaf	*Althaea officinalis* L.
Marshmallow root	*Althaea officinalis* L.
Maté, Paraguay tea	*Ilex paraguariensis* ST.-HIL.
Meadowsweet flower, herb	*Filipendula ulmaria* var. *vulgare* (L.) MAXIM.
Melilot, king's clover	*Melilotus officinalis* (L.) PALL., *M. altissima* THIULL.
Milk thistle, St. Mary's thistle	*Silybum marianum* L. (GAERTN.)
Mint oil	*Mentha arvensis* L. var. *piperascens* MALINV.
Motherwort, lion's tail	*Leonurus cardiaca* L.
Mugwort, common wormwood	*Artemisia vulgaris* L.
Mullein flower, verbascum flower	*Verbascum densiflorum* BERTOL., *V. phlomoides* L.
Myrrh, myrrh tincture	*Commiphora myrrha* (NEES) ENGLER
Neem	*Azadirachta indica* A. JUSS (syn. *Antelaea azadirachta* L.)
Nettle leaf, herb	*Urtica dioica* L., *U. urens* L.
Nettle root	*Urtica dioica* L., *U. urens* L.

Oak bark	*Quercus robur* L.
Oat straw	*Avena sativa* L.
Olive leaf	*Olea europaea* L.
Olive oil	*Olea europaea* L.
Onion	*Allium cepa* L.
Parsley herb, root	*Petroselinum crispum* (MILL.) NYM.
Passion flower herb, maypop	*Passiflora incarnata* L.
Peppermint leaf	*Mentha × piperita* L.
Peppermint oil	*Mentha × piperita* L.
Petasitis, butterbur	*Petasites hybridus* (L.) GAERTN., MEY. & SCHERB
Podophyllum, mayapple, American mandrake	*Podophyllum peltatum* L.
Pokeweed, phytolacca	*Phytolacca americana* L.
Pollen	Pollinae
Poplar bud	*Populus tremula* L.
Poplar leaf, bark	*Populus tremula* L.
Primula flower, root; cowslip flower, root	*Primula veris* L.
Pumpkin seed	*Cucurbita pepo* L.
Puncture vine, burra gokhru	*Tribulus terrestris* L.
Pygeum	*Pygeum africanum* HOOK F. (syn. *Prunus africana* (HOOK. f.) KALKMAN)
Pyrethrum flower, Dalmatian insect flower	*Tanacetum cinerariifolium* (TREVIR.) SCH. BIP.
Raspberry leaf	*Rubus idaeus* L.
Red clover	*Trifolium pratense* L.
Restharrow, cammock	*Ononis spinosa* L.
Rhatany root, Peruvian rhatany	*Krameria lappacea* (DOMB.) BURD. et SIMP. (syn. *K. triandra* RUIZ et PAV.)
Rhubarb root	*Rheum palmatum* L., *R. officinale* BAILL.
Roman chamomile, English chamomile	*Chamaemelum nobile* (L.) ALL.
Rose hips, dog rose	*Rosa canina* L., *R. pendulina* L.
Rosemary leaf	*Rosmarinus officinalis* L.
Saffron	*Crocus sativus* L.
Sage, red sage	*Salvia officinalis* L.
Sandalwood	*Santalum album* L.
Sarsaparilla	*Smilax* spp.
Sassafras	*Sassafras albidum* (NUTT.) NEES
Saw palmetto	*Serenoa repens* (BARTR.) SMALL
Schisandra	*Schisandra chinensis* (TURCZ.) BAILL.

Seneca root, senega root, snakeroot, rattlesnake root	*Polygala senega* L.
Senna	*Cassia senna* L., *C. angustifolia* VAHL.
Senna pod	*Cassia senna* L. (syn. *C. acutifolia* DEL.), *C. angustifolia* VAHL.
Shepherd's purse, caseweed herb	*Capsella bursa-pastoris* (L.) MEDIK.
Silverweed, goose gras	*Potentilla anserina* L.
Slippery elm bark	*Ulmus rubra* MÜHLENB.
Small-flowered willow herb	*Epilobium parviflorum* SCHREB.
Soybean lecithin	*Glycine max* (L.) MERR.
Spanish psyllium seed, French psyllium seed	*Plantago afra* L.
Spearmint leaf	*Mentha spicata* L. spp. *spicata*
Speedwell	*Veronica officinalis* L.
St. John's wort	*Hypericum perforatum* L.
Tea tree oil	*Melaleuca alternifolia* CHEEL.
Temoe lawak, Javanese turmeric	*Curcuma xanthorrhiza* ROXB.
Thuja, arborvitae	*Thuja occidentalis* L.
Thyme	*Thymus vulgaris* L., *T. zygis* L.
Tormentil	*Potentilla erecta* (L.) RÄUSCH.
Turmeric	*Curcuma domestica* VAL. (syn. *C. longa* L.)
Uzara root	*Xysmalobium undulatum* (L.) R. BR.
Valerian root, tincture	*Valeriana officinalis* L.
Vervain	*Verbena officinalis* L.
Walnut leaf	*Juglans regia* L.
White dead nettle, archangel	*Lamium album* L.
Wild thyme, mother of thyme, serpyllum	*Thymus serpyllum* L.
Willow bark	*Salix purpurea* L., *S. daphnoides* VIL. (among others)
Witch hazel bark, hamamelis bark	*Hamamelis virginiana* L.
Witch hazel leaf, hamamelis leaf	*Hamamelis virginiana* L.
Wormwood, absinthe	*Artemisia absinthium* L.
Yarrow, milfoil	*Achillea millefolium* L.
Yellow bedstraw herb, lady's bedstraw	*Galium verum* L.
Yellow chaste weed, everlasting flower	*Helichrysum arenarium* (L.) MOENCH
Yohimbe	*Pausinystalia yohimbe* (K. SCHUM.) PIERRE ex BEILLE
Zedoary	*Curcuma zedoaria* (CHRISTM.) ROSC.

LATIN-ENGLISH

Achillea millefolium L.	Yarrow, milfoil
Acorus calamus L.	Calamus, sweet flag
Aesculus hippocastanum L.	Horse chestnut seed
Agrimonia eupatoria L.	Agrimony
Agropyron repens (L.) P. BEAUV.	Couch grass, quack grass
Alchemilla xanthochlora ROTHM.	Lady's mantle, lion's foot
Allium cepa L.	Onion
Allium sativum L.	Garlic, garlic oil
Aloe barbadensis MILL.	Barbados aloe, Curaçao aloe
Aloe ferox MILL.	Cape aloe
Alpinia officinarum HANCE	Galangal, Chinese ginger, galanga
Althaea officinalis L.	Marshmallow leaf
Althaea officinalis L.	Marshmallow root
Ammi visnaga (L.) LAM.	Khella, visnaga
Anethum graveolens L. ssp. *graveolens*	Dill
Angelica archangelica L.	Angelica root, European angelica root
Angelica sinensis (OLIV.) DIELS	Dong quai, danggui
Arctium lappa L.	Burdock, great burdock
Arctostaphylos uva-ursi (L.) SPRENGEL	Bearberry leaf
Arnica montana L.	Arnica flower, leopard's bane
Artemisia absinthium L.	Wormwood, absinthe
Artemisia vulgaris L.	Mugwort, common wormwood
Astragalus membranaceus (FISCH.) BGE. var. *mongolicus* (BGE.) HSIAO	Astragalus
Avena sativa L.	Oat straw
Azadirachta indica A. JUSS (syn. *Antelaea azadirachta* L.)	Neem
Betula pubescens EHRH., *B. pendula* ROTH.	Birch leaf
Boswellia carteri BIRDW.	Indian frankincense
Boswellia serrata ROXB. ex COLEBR.	Indian olibanum tree
Calendula officinalis L.	Calendula, marigold flower
Capsella bursa-pastoris (L.) MEDIK.	Shepherd's purse, caseweed herb
Capsicum frutescens L.	Cayenne pepper, chilies, tabasco pepper

Carlina acaulis L.	Carline thistle
Carum carvi L.	Caraway
Cassia senna L.,	Senna
C. angustifolia VAHL.	
Cassia senna L. (syn.	Senna pod
C. acutifolia DEL.),	
C. angustifolia VAHL.	
Centaurium erythraea RAFN.	Common centaury, centaury herb
Cetraria islandica (L.) ACH.	Iceland moss
Chamaemelum nobile	Roman chamomile, English chamomile
(L.) ALL.	
Chelidonium majus L.	Greater celandine
Cichorium intybus L.	Chicory, succory
Cimicifuga racemosa	Black cohosh
(L.) NUTT.	
Cinnamomum aromaticum	Chinese cassia/cassia
NEES.	
Cinnamomum ceylanicum	Cinnamon bark, Ceylon cinnamon
BLUME, *C. verum* J. S.	
PRESL.	
Citrus aurantium L.	Bitter orange peel
ssp. *aurantium*	
Cnicus benedictus L.	Blessed thistle, holy thistle
Commiphora mukul	Guggul, guggal
(HOOK. ex STOCKS)	
ENGL.	
Commiphora myrrha	Myrrh, myrrh tincture
(NEES) ENGLER	
Coriandrum sativum L.	Coriander
Crataegus monogyna JAQC.	Hawthorn herb with flower; haw, white thorn
Crocus sativus L.	Saffron
Cucurbita pepo L.	Pumpkin seed
Curcuma domestica VAL.	Turmeric
(syn. *C. longa* L.)	
Curcuma xanthorrhiza	Temoe lawak, Javanese turmeric
ROXB.	
Curcuma zedoaria	Zedoary
(CHRISTM.) ROSC.	
Cymbopogon winterianus	Java citronella oil
IOWITT.	
Cynara scolymus L.	Artichoke leaf
Drosera madagascariensis	Drosera, sundew herb
DC., *D. peltata* SMITH	
Echinacea pallida (NUTT.)	Echinacea pallida root
NUTT.	

Echinacea purpurea (L.) MOENCH	Echinacea purpurea herb
Elettaria cardamomum (L.) MATON	Cardamom
Eleutherococcus senticosus MAXIM.	Eleuthero, Siberian ginseng
Ephedra sinica STAPF, *E. shennungiana* TANG	Ephedra herb, ma huang
Epilobium parviflorum SCHREB.	Small-flowered willow herb
Epimedium spp.	Horny goat weed, barrenwort
Equisetum arvense L.	Horsetail
Eucalyptus globulus LABILL.	Eucalyptus
Eucalyptus globulus LABILL.	Eucalyptus oil
Euprasia stricta WOLFF ex. J. F. LEHM.	Eyebright herb
Fagopyrum esculentum MOENCH	Buckwheat herb
Filipendula ulmaria var. *vulgare* (L.) MAXIM.	Meadowsweet flower, herb
Foeniculum vulgare MILL., var. *vulgare,* var. *dulce*	Fennel
Frangula purshiana (DC.) COOP.	Cascara sagrada, sacred bark, chittem bark
Fraxinus ornus L.	Manna
Fucus vesiculosus L.	Fucus, kelp
Fumaria officinalis L.	Fumitory herb, earth smoke
Galeopsis segetum NECKER	Hemp nettle
Galium verum L.	Yellow bedstraw herb, lady's bedstraw
Gentiana lutea L.	Gentian
Ginkgo biloba L.	Ginkgo, ginkgo biloba extract
Glycine max (L.) MERR.	Soybean lecithin
Glycyrrhiza glabra L.	Licorice root, glycyrrhiza
Graminaceae, meadow flowers	Hayseed flower
Hamamelis virginiana L.	Witch hazel bark, hamamelis bark
Hamamelis virginiana L.	Witch hazel leaf, hamamelis leaf
Harpagophytum procumbens (BURCH.) DC.	Devil's claw
Harungana madagascariensis LAM. ex POIR.	Haronga, harungana bark, leaf
Hedera helix L.	Ivy, English ivy
Helichrysum arenarium (L.) MOENCH	Yellow chaste weed, everlasting flower

Herniaria glabra L.	Herniary, rupturewort
Hibiscus sabdariffa L.	Hibiscus flower, Jamaica sorrel, roselle
Humulus lupulus L.	Hops
Hydrastis canadensis L.	Goldenseal, hydrastis
Hypericum perforatum L.	St. John's wort
Ilex paraguariensis ST.-HIL.	Maté, Paraguay tea
Juglans regia L.	Walnut leaf
Juniperus communis L.	Juniper berry
Krameria lappacea (DOMB.) BURD. et SIMP. (syn. *K. triandra* RUIZ et PAV.)	Rhatany root, Peruvian rhatany
Lamium album L.	White dead nettle, archangel
Lavandula angustifolia MILL.	Lavender flower
Lavandula angustifolia MILL.	Lavender oil
Lawsonia inermis L.	Henna
Leonurus cardiaca L.	Motherwort, lion's tail
Levisticum officinale KOCH	Lovage root
Linum usitatissimum L.	Linseed, flaxseed
Lycopodium clavatum L.	Lycopodium herb, club moss
Lycopus europaeus L., *L. virginicus* L.	Bugleweed, gypsywort
Malva neglecta WALLR., *Malve sylvestris* ssp. *mauritiana* (L.) BOISS. ex COUT	Mallow leaf and flower
Marrubium vulgare L.	Horehound, hoarhound
Marsdenia cundurango Reich. f.	Cundurango, eagle vine
Matricaria recutita L.	Chamomile, German chamomile flower
Melaleuca alternifolia CHEEL.	Tea tree oil
Melilotus officinalis (L.) PALL., *M. altissima* THIULL.	Melilot, king's clover
Melissa officinalis L.	Balm leaf, lemon balm, melissa
Mentha arvensis L. var. *piperascens* MALINV.	Mint oil
Mentha × *piperita* L.	Peppermint leaf
Mentha × *piperita* L.	Peppermint oil
Mentha spicata L. spp. *spicata*	Spearmint leaf
Menyanthes trifoliata L.	Buckbean, bogbean
Olea europaea L.	Olive leaf

Olea europaea L.	Olive oil
Ononis spinosa L.	Restharrow, cammock
Orthosiphon aristatus (BLUME) MIQ.	Java tea
Panax ginseng C. A. MEY.	Chinese or Korean ginseng root
Passiflora incarnata L.	Passion flower herb, maypop
Pausinystalia yohimbe (K. SCHUM.) PIERRE ex BEILLE	Yohimbe
Persea americana MILL.	Avocado oil
Petasites hybridus (L.) GAERTN., MEY. & SCHERB	Petasitis, butterbur
Petroselinum crispum (MILL.) NYM.	Parsley herb, root
Peumus boldus MOL.	Boldo leaf
Phytolacca americana L.	Pokeweed, phytolacca
Pimpinella anisum L.	Anise, aniseed
Pimpinella major (L.) HUDS., *P. saxifraga* L.	Great burnet saxifrage, saxifrage
Plantago afra L.	Spanish psyllium seed, French psyllium seed
Plantago lanceolata L.	English plantain, ribwort
Plantago ovata FORSK.	Blond psyllium husk/seed, Indian plantago, ispaghula
Podophyllum peltatum L.	Podophyllum, mayapple, American mandrake
Pollinae	Pollen
Polygala senega L.	Seneca root, senega root, snakeroot, rattlesnake root
Polygonum aviculare L.	Black knotweed, hogweed
Populus tremula L.	Poplar bud
Populus tremula L.	Poplar leaf, bark
Potentilla anserina L.	Silverweed, goose gras
Potentilla erecta (L.) RÄUSCH.	Tormentil
Primula veris L.	Primula flower, root; cowslip flower, root
Prunus spinosa L.	Blackthorn flower
Prunus spinosa L.	Blackthorn fruit
Psychotria ipecacuanha (BROT.) STOKES	Ipecacuanha root, ipecac
Pygeum africanum (HOOK.) F. (syn. *Prunus africana* (HOOK. f.) KALKMAN)	Pygeum
Quercus robur L.	Oak bark
Rhamnus cathartica L.	Buckthorn
Rhamnus frangula L.	Frangula bark, buckthorn bark
Rheum palmatum L., *R. officinale* BAILL.	Rhubarb root

Rosa canina L., *R. pendulina* L.	Rose hips, dog rose
Rosmarinus officinalis L.	Rosemary leaf
Rubus fruticosus L.	Blackberry leaf
Rubus idaeus L.	Raspberry leaf
Ruscus aculeatus L.	Butcher's-broom, box holly

Salix purpurea L.,
   S. daphnoides VIL.
   (among others)
	Willow bark

Salvia officinalis L.	Sage, red sage
Salvia triloba L. FIL.	Greek sage leaf
Sambucus nigra L.	Black or European elder flower
Santalum album L.	Sandalwood
Sassafras albidum (NUTT.) NEES	Sassafras
Schisandra chinensis (TURCZ.) BAILL.	Schisandra
Serenoa repens (BARTR.) SMALL	Saw palmetto
Silybum marianum L. (GAERTN.)	Milk thistle, St. Mary's thistle
Smilax spp.	Sarsaparilla
Solidago gigantea AIT. ssp. *gigantea*	Early goldenrod
Solidago virgaurea L.	European goldenrod
Symphytum officinale L.	Comfrey leaf, herb
Symphytum officinale L.	Comfrey root
Syzygium aromaticum (L.) MERR. et L. M. PERRY	Cloves, clove oil

Tanacetum
   cinerariifolium (TREVIR.)
   SCH. BIP.
	Pyrethrum flower, Dalmatian insect flower

Tanacetum parthenium (L.) SCHULTZ BIP.	Feverfew herb
Taraxacum officinale WEB.	Dandelion root and herb
Thuja occidentalis L.	Thuja, arborvitae
Thymus serpyllum L.	Wild thyme, mother of thyme, serpyllum
Thymus vulgaris L., *T. zygis* L.	Thyme

Tilia cordata MILL.,
   T. platyphyllos SCOP.,
   T. vulgaris HEYNE
	Linden flower, lime tree flower

Tribulus terrestris L.	Puncture vine, burra gokhru
Trifolium pratense L.	Red clover

Trigonella foenum-graecum L.	Fenugreek seed
Turnera diffusa WILLD. ex SCHULT. ssp. *gigantea, Turnera diffusa* var. *aphrodisiaca* (KINGDON-WARD) URBAN	Damiana
Tussilago farfara L.	Coltsfoot leaf, tussilago leaf
Ulmus rubra MÜHLENB.	Slippery elm bark
Uncaria tomentosa (WILLD.) DC.	Cat's claw, uña de gato
Urtica dioica L., *U. urens* L.	Nettle leaf, herb
Urtica dioica L., *U. urens* L.	Nettle root
Vaccinium myrtillus L.	Bilberry, blueberry
Vaccinium myrtillus L.	Bilberry leaf, blueberry leaf
Valeriana officinalis L.	Valerian root, tincture
Verbascum densiflorum L. BERTOL., *V. phlomoides* L.	Mullein flower, verbascum flower
Verbena officinalis L.	Vervain
Veronica officinalis L.	Speedwell
Viola tricolor L.	Heartsease, wild pansy
Viscum album L.	European mistletoe
Vitex agnus-castus L.	Chaste tree
Vitis vinifera L.	Grape seed
Withania somnifera DUNAL	Ashwagandha
Xysmalobium undulatum (L.) R. BR.	Uzara root
Zea mays L.	Corn silk
Zingiber officinale ROSC.	Ginger, ginger root

Bibliography

Official Literature

Braun, R. (Ed.) (2003). *Standardzulassungen für Fertigarzneimittel,* basic issue including fifteenth supplement, Deutscher Apotheker Verlag, Stuttgart; Govi Verlag, Eschborn.

Commission E-Monographs: Aufbereitungsmonographien der phytotherapeutischen Therapierichtung und Stoffgruppe, DAV-Software PharmaMed (CD-ROM), Deutscher Apotheker Verlag, Stuttgart.

Deutscher Arzneimittel Codex (1986, including Supplement 2003). Deutscher Apotheker Verlag, Stuttgart; Govi Verlag, Eschborn.

Deutsches Arzneibuch Kommentar (DAB 2003). Deutscher Apotheker Verlag, Stuttgart; Govi Verlag, Eschborn.

ESCOP-Monographs (2004). *Official Monographs of the European Scientific Co-operation on Phytotherapy,* Argyle House, Gandy Street, UK-Devon, EX 43 LF.

Pharmacopoea Europaea 4 (2003). *Commentary,* Deutscher Apotheker Verlag, Stuttgart; Govi Verlag, Eschborn.

Reference Books

Benedum, J., Loew, D., and Schilcher, H. (1984). *Arzneipflanzen in der Traitionellen Medizin,* Second Edition, Kooperation Phyto-therapie, Krahe Druck, Unkel.

Bisset, Norman G. and Wichtl, Max (Eds.) (2001). *Herbal Drugs and Phytopharmaceuticals: A Handbook for Practice on a Scientific Basis,* Medpharm Scientific Publishers, Stuttgart; CRC Press, Boca Raton, FL.

Blaschek, W., Ebel, S., Hackenthal, E., Holzgrabe, U., Keller, K., and Reichling, J. (Eds.) (2001). *Hager ROM, Hagers Handbuch der Drogen und Arzneistoffe,* Springer electronic media, Springer Verlag, Berlin, New York.

Blaschek, W., Hänsel, R., Keller, K., Reichling, J., Rimpler, H., and Schneider, G. (Eds.) (1998). *Hagers Handbuch der Pharmazeutischen Praxis:* Fifth Edition, supplements 2 and 3, Springer Verlag, Berlin, New York.

Brendler, T., Grünwald, J., and Jänicke, C. (Eds.) (2003). *Herb-CD 5—Herbal Remedies,* English/German, Medpharm Scientific Publishers, Stuttgart.

Brinkmann, H., Wißmeyer, K., Gehrmann, B., Koch, W.-G., Tschirch, C. (2004). *Phytotherapie,* Wissenschaftliche Verlagsgesellschaft, Stuttgart.

Chang, H. M. and But, P. P.-H. (Eds.) (1986). *Pharmacology and Applications of Chinese Materia Medica,* Yao, S.-Ch., Wang, L.-L., and Yeung S. C.-S. (transl.), Volume I, World Scientific Publishing Co Pte Ltd., Singapore.

Chang, H. M., Yeung, H. W., Tso, W.-W., and Koo, A. (Eds.) (1985). *Advances in Chinese Medicinal Materials Research,* World Scientific Publishing Co Pte Ltd., Singapore.

Dingermann, T., Hänsel, R., and Zündorf, I. (2003). *Pharmazeutische Biologie,* Springer Verlag, Berlin, New York.

Dingermann, T. and Loew, D. (2003). *Phytopharmakologie,* Wissenschaftliche Verlagsgesellschaft, Stuttgart.

Erhardt, W., Götz, E., Bödecker, N., and Seybold, S. (2002). *Zander Dictionary of Plant Names,* Seventeenth Edition, Verlag Eugen Ulmer, Stuttgart.

Frohne, D. (2002). *Heilpflanzenlexikon,* Seventh Edition, Wissenschaftliche Verlagsgesellschaft, Stuttgart.

Frohne, D. and Pfänder, H. J. (1997). *Giftpflanzen,* Fourth Edition, Wissenschaftliche Verlagsgesellschaft, Stuttgart.

Fugmann, B., Lang-Fugmann, S., and Steglich, M. (Eds.), (1997). *Römpp Lexikon der Chemie, Vol. Naturstoffe,* Georg Thieme Verlag, Stuttgart.

Gehrmann, B., Koch, W.-G., Tschirch, C. O., and Brinkmann, H. (2000). *Arzneidrogenprofile,* Deutscher Apotheker Verlag, Stuttgart.

Grieve F.R.H.S., M. (1971). *A Modern Herbal,* Revised Edition, Barnes and Noble Inc., New York.

Hänsel, R. (1991). *Phytopharmaka,* Second Edition, Springer Verlag, Berlin, New York.

Hänsel, R., Keller, K., Rimpler, H., and Schneider, G. (Eds.) (1992-1994). *Hagers Handbuch der Pharmazeutischen Praxis,* Fifth Edition, Volumes 4-6, Springer Verlag, Berlin, New York.

Hänsel, R., Sticher, O., and Steinegger, E. (1999). *Pharmakognosie—Phytopharmazie,* Sixth Edition, Springer Verlag, Berlin, New York. Haffner, F., Schultz, O. E., Schmid, W., and Braun, R. (1997). *Normdosen gebräuchlicher Arzneistoffe und Drogen,* Ninth Edition, Wissenschaftliche Verlagsgesellschaft, Stuttgart.

Hiller, K. and Melzig, M. F. (1999). *Lexikon der Arzneipflanzen und Drogen,* Volumes A-K, L-Z, Spektrum Akademischer Verlag, Heidelberg, Berlin.

Hoppe, H. A. (1975-1987). *Drogenkunde,* Eighth Edition, Volumes 1-3, W. de Gruyter Verlag, Berlin.

Jänicke, C., Grünwald, J., and Brendler, T. (2003). *Handbuch Phytotherapie,* Wissenschaftliche Verlagsgesellschaft, Stuttgart.

Loew, D. and Rietbrock, N. (Eds.) (1995-2002). *Phytopharmaka in Forschung und klinischer Anwendung,* Volumes 1-7, Steinkopff Verlag, Darmstadt.

Madaus, G. (1987). *Lehrbuch der Biologischen Heilmittel,* Volumes 1-11, Mediamed Verlag, Ravensburg. Reprint of the Ed. Leipzig 1938.

Meyer-Buchtela, E. (1999). *Tee-Rezepturen,* basic issue with first supplement, Wissenschaftliche Veragsgesellschaft, Stuttgart.